Thieme

Advanced Techniques in Oriental Medicine

Skya Abbate, MA, DOM, Dipl Ac, Dipl CH

Department of Clinical Medicine
Southwest Acupuncture College
Santa Fe/Albuquerque New Mexico and Boulder
Colorado, USA

Foreword by Giovanni Maciocia

34 illustrations
33 tables

Georg Thieme Verlag
Stuttgart · New York

Library of Congress Cataloging-in-Publication Data

Abbate, Skya.
Taming the tiger: advanced techniques
in Oriental medicine/Skya Abbate.
p.; cm.
Includes bibliographical references and index.
ISBN 3-13-143051-6 (GTV: alk. paper)
ISBN 1-58890-493-8 (TNY: alk paper)
1. Medicine, Oriental. I. Title.
[DNLM: 1. Medicine, Oriental Traditional.
2. Acupuncture Therapy. WB 50.1 A123t 2006]
610–dc22 200613393

Photos by Dr. Anthony Abbate, DOM
Santa Fe, New Mexico, USA; with the exception
of Figs. 1.2, 1.2, 4.1 and 13.1 provided by Seirin Europe/
3B Scientific, Hamburg, Germany

Illustrations by Jaye Oliver, Santa Fe, New Mexico, USA

Rüdigerstrasse 14, 70469 Stuttgart, Germany
http://www.thieme.de
Thieme New York, 333 Seventh Avenue,
New York, NY 10001, USA
http://www.thieme.com

Typesetting by Sommer Druck, Feuchtwangen
Printed in Germany by Grafisches Centrum Cuno, Calbe
10-ISBN 3-13-143051-6 (GTV)
13-ISBN 978-3-13-143051-9 (GTV)
10-ISBN 1-58890-493-8 (TNY)
13-ISBN 978-1-58890-493-5 (TNY) 1 2 3 4 5 6

Blood and *qi* are a human's spirit. It is not all right to not be careful in nourishing them.

"Treatise of the Eight Righteous Brilliances" in the *Su Wen* (*Simple Questions*)

Dedication

To all those who work in the healthcare professions, especially those who selflessly care for the sick and the poor.

To Father Vidal Martinez for always reminding me to pray for the sick.

Acknowledgement

To my husband, Anthony, for always believing in my ability to write a textbook and for giving me the leisure to devote my time to writing.

All money derived from the sale of this book will be donated to the Missionary Oblates of Mary Immaculate.

Preface

> When caring for a patient, concentrate on the situation without being distracted by the circumstances, as if standing on the brink of a gorge not wanting to fall in. When you grasp the needle, do so with great care, firm strength and caution for the peril, as if holding a tiger's tail: one wrong move and great harm could befall.
>
> *Huang Di Nei Jing*

Ten years ago, my first textbook, *Holding the Tiger's Tail: An Acupuncture Techniques Manual in the Treatment of Disease*, was published. Since then that book has been used in many acupuncture colleges both in the United States and Europe as a beginners-to-intermediate textbook for acupuncture students and practitioners. Following that book, two specialized texts were published, a Japanese treatment book, *The Art of Palpatory Diagnosis in Oriental Medicine* both in English and Italian (Churchill Livingstone, 2001 and 2004 respectively), and a Chinese ear acupuncture book, *Chinese Auricular Acupuncture* (CRC Press, 2004).

As my final needle techniques book, *Advanced Techniques in Oriental Medicine*, this text covers more advanced skills in Oriental medicine with an emphasis on needle technique within the context of treating common illnesses. A section on adjunct therapies for the Oriental medical practitioner is also included.

The body of knowledge of Oriental medicine is elegantly simple, and easy to understand, and to diagnose and treat with the needle and supporting modalities. Students and practitioners of Oriental medicine know the power of Oriental medicine as a diagnostic and treatment style. Most practitioners start off their practice learning all the treatment of disease (or differentiation of disease) protocols in the books available at the time of graduation, or strategies learned from experienced instructors. How we end up treating in our clinical career is a function both of our interests or specialties, as well as the disorders of the patients who come to our door. However, treatments do not need to be long, complex, employ many needles, and of course, need not be painful. As in most things in life, what are requisite to treatment are clarity, consciousness, compassion, and kindness.

I hope these simple yet effective treatment strategies will allow you to deliver effective healthcare to those in distress and to increase your satisfaction with your practice by "taming the tiger," through the mastery of the needle and the tools of Oriental medicine.

Skya Abbate
2006

Foreword

When comparing acupuncture to Chinese herbal medicine, it is often said that the latter is more difficult to learn and to practice. I tend to disagree. Acupuncture is probably more difficult to learn and to practice because it involves so many variables.

To give an effective treatment, there are certain steps that are common to both acupuncture and herbal medicine, i.e.:

- a correct diagnosis (whatever system or type of Oriental medicine is used)
- a correct treatment principle
- a correct choice of treatment.

With herbal medicine, if the diagnosis and treatment principle are both correct, the prescription practically picks itself because of the close identification of treatment principle with categories of prescriptions. For example, when we say that the treatment principle is to clear heat and cool blood we mean that we need to clear heat at the blood level: this automatically corresponds to the category of cooling blood prescriptions. Similarly, when we say that we need to resolve toxic heat it means that we need to choose a formula from the category of prescriptions that resolve toxic heat.

With acupuncture, the correspondence between treatment principle and choice of treatment is not as rigid or unequivocal. For example, there are only a few points that specifically cool blood (e.g., PC-3 *qu ze*). Therefore, cooling blood with acupuncture is achieved in a different way and without such a straightforward correspondence between treatment principle and categories of formulae as in Chinese herbal medicine.

The modality of working with acupuncture is profoundly different to that of Chinese herbal medicine. Chinese herbal medicine is based on the use of drugs of plant origin. These work in a different way to, and are intrinsically safer than drugs; however, they are drugs nevertheless. They contain active principles that affect the body's physiology in a similar way to drugs. For example, to resolve edema with Chinese herbal medicine we may choose the formula *Wu Ling San*, which contains herbs that are diuretic and resolve edema by stimulating urination.

Acupuncture works in a completely different way because it essentially works only by regulating *qi*. In contrast to herbal medicine, how can acupuncture resolve edema? How can we stimulate urination with acupuncture? Acupuncture can resolve edema only by regulating the ascending/descending and entering/exiting of *qi* in the water passages of the three burners.

When compared to herbal medicine, therefore, the acupuncture treatment is not rigidly determined by the treatment principle, and the choice of points is much more flexible.

Another important difference is that acupuncture is more subject to cosmic influences than herbal medicine. By that I mean that, being based on manipulation of a subtle energy such as *qi*, acupuncture is more subject to influences of the time of day, season, moon phase, the menstrual cycle in women, etc. For example, in an article in a Chinese medicine journal Dr. Chen Ming treated 43 patients with asthma by giving them acupuncture during specific solar terms and compared the results to those in 24 patients treated not according to solar terms.[1]

The solar terms are 24 periods of 2 weeks each in a year, beginning from the first day of the Chinese New Year (which would fall on a different date of the Western calendar each year). The solar terms during which the treatment was administered were:

- Spring Equinox (4th solar term)
- Summer Solstice (10th solar term)
- Autumn Equinox (16th solar term)
- Winter Solstice (22nd solar term).

The FEV (Forced Expiratory Volume) was measured in each patient in each group, and the patients treated according to the solar terms regis-

[1] Chen Ming Preliminary Study on the Relationship between Acupuncture in Different Solar Terms and Changes in Pulmonary Function in Asthma in Chinese Acupuncture and Moxibustion. *Zhong Guo Zhen Jiu.* 2000;20(3):155.

tered a better improvement than those who were not.

The fact that acupuncture is subject to cosmic cycles is probably the reason why a patient never reacts in the same way when we apply exactly the same treatment. For many years I have noticed over and over again that when a patient has a very positive reaction to a particular acupuncture treatment, the reaction is *never* the same when we repeat that treatment.

After deciding on a treatment principle, an acupuncture treatment is subject to many more variables than herbal medicine. In fact, after choosing a treatment principle, we still need to work out a suitable point combination that takes into account many factors, such as the actions of the points in relation to the pattern treated, the harmonious combination of points, the time of day, season, and even moon phase.

In fact, when choosing points for an acupuncture treatment there are two different considerations:

- the selection of points according to their action
- the combination of points according to channel dynamics.

Acupuncture works via the channels, not just via isolated points, so that each point should not only be considered for its individual action but also for its place within the channel system. Even if we master the action of each individual point, this is still not enough to give an effective acupuncture treatment, as each point must be seen within the dynamics of the channel system so as to attain a harmonious combination of points.

The balance of the point combination is essential to the success of an acupuncture treatment. Indeed, a balanced point combination is as important to the therapeutic result as the needling technique. The latter is, of course, very important to the success of an acupuncture treatment but the harmonious combination of points is often overlooked: they are both important because they reflect two different viewpoints. In a way, the stress placed on needling technique is based on a point-centered view of acupuncture, while the stress placed on the combination of points is based on a channel-centered view of acupuncture. Both these viewpoints are important and both need to be taken into account.

When giving an acupuncture treatment, there are very many practical variables, such as a correct point location, correct needling direction and depth, correct obtaining of *de qi*, and correct needling manipulation. In addition, more variables are introduced when moxa is considered: Should we use moxa? On which point? Which type of moxibustion?

For all the above reasons, I think that acupuncture is very difficult to practice: it is indeed an art. There are comparatively few books that deal with the techniques of acupuncture in a detailed and practical way. *Advanced Techniques in Oriental Medicine* is such a book, which makes it so welcome to students and practitioners of acupuncture, whatever the style practiced.

Dr. Skya Abbate is uniquely placed to introduce the reader to the complexities of acupuncture as she has long experience both as a practitioner and a clinical teacher. She is therefore aware of the needs of students and practitioners. Dr. Abbate's clinical and teaching experience is apparent in every page of the book.

The transmission of a medical tradition from one culture to another is always fraught with difficulties. When transmitting a medical system between two such different cultures as the ancient Chinese and modern Western cultures, the difficulties are even greater. I personally feel we should strike a balance between adhering firmly to the tradition and adapting this tradition to the needs of Western students and patients. Adhering rigidly and blindingly to tradition will not serve the needs of our patients, while adapting a medical system without fully understanding it first may create theories which have no basis in practice.

Dr. Abbate's book strikes such a balance as it presents the traditional techniques of acupuncture and creatively adapts them to the needs of Western patients. For example, there is an innovative and important chapter on the treatment of the spirit with acupuncture. She correlates spirit treatment with treatment of the blood level.

Dr. Abbate's book is an example of the kind of books needed to ensure a faithful and creative transmission of Chinese medicine to the West.

Giovanni Maciocia

About the Author

Skya Abbate, MA, DOM., Dipl Ac, Dipl CH, began her career as a medical sociologist serving as a Peace Corps volunteer in Brazil, and then later taught in the Sociology Department of the University of Rhode Island (1978–81). She holds a BA in Sociology from Salve Regina College (Newport, RI 1973) where she graduated summa cum laude and class valedictorian, and an MA in Sociology from the University of Rhode Island (1978).

Following pre-med studies at the University of Rhode Island, in 1983, Skya graduated from the acupuncture program of the Institute of Traditional Medicine in Santa Fe, NM. She then undertook two advanced clinical training programs with the Academy of Traditional Chinese Medicine in Beijing, China in 1988 and 1989.

Skya is a licensed Doctor of Oriental Medicine in the State of New Mexico, Executive Director of Southwest Acupuncture College with three campuses in Santa Fe and Albuquerque, NM and Boulder, CO. She was former President of the New Mexico Association of Acupuncture and Oriental Medicine and has served for over 6 years as an educational expert and Commissioner for the Accreditation Commission for Acupuncture and Oriental Medicine (ACAOM), the national organization that accredits professional degree programs in Oriental medicine.

Skya is the author of four additional books: *Beijing: The New Forbidden City* (Southwest Acupuncture College Press, 1991), *Holding the Tiger's Tail: An Acupuncture Techniques Manual in the Treatment of Disease* (Southwest Acupuncture College Press, 1996), *The Art of Palpatory Diagnosis in Oriental Medicine* (Churchill Livingstone, 2001) also published in Italian in 2004 as *Palpazione Diagnostica in Medicina Orientale*, and *Chinese Auricular Medicine* (CRC Press, 2004). She has authored over 36 journal articles published in such prestigious journals as the *American Journal of Acupuncture*, the *Journal of Chinese Medicine*, the *New England Journal of Traditional Chinese Medicine*, and *Acupuncture Today* where she served for 6 years as the needle technique columnist. Two final texts are in progress—*The Spiritual Practice of Clinical Medicine*, and a point location and energetics book, along with a book of poetry and numerous Catholic inspirational short stories. Her scholarship and knowledge of the field has made her a sought-after book proposal reviewer for Elsevier, Taylor and Francis, Mosby and other medical publishers. With over 20 years of private practice experience and teaching she is one of the most qualified, respected, and prolific writers in Oriental medicine in the Western world.

Skya teaches needle technique, diagnosis, and Japanese acupuncture systems at Southwest Acupuncture College. She also has a private practice integrating classical Chinese treatment with her sub-specialty in Japanese acupuncture.

Contents

I General Approaches to Treatment

II The Treatment of Specific Diseases

III Other Modalities—Treatment Tools Complementary to Acupuncture

IV Specialized Use of Points

Appendix

I General Approaches to Treatment

1 The Needle

As the *Ling Shu*, the second part of the *Huang Di Nei Jing*, the 2000-year old book on traditional acupuncture, posits, "If you should want to treat illness there is nothing so good as the needle" and certainly, the needle is the primary tool of treatment for the acupuncturist. Ironically though, in my experience as a teacher, I have found students to be disinterested in the specifics of the needle, such as its gauge and length, and are more interested in actually using it. This is understandable in the sense that in their passion for the medicine and compassion for the patient they are anxious to help alleviate suffering.

While I am sure that the students do learn this material in school, I also know that it is not given the pre-eminence it deserves, nor are the students held accountable for it over other topics. This relative lack of basic, fundamental training can easily be rectified if students are taught the facts with the proper attention and respect the subject deserves. As a result of my observations as an advanced needle technique instructor therefore, it would be wise to take some time to review the various parameters of the needle over the needling process. Correct understanding of the gauges and lengths of needles contributes to their correct usage and thus clinical success.

■ Needle Composition and Safety

According to anthropological data, ancient needles were made of bamboo, stone, and steel. Modern day needles are made out of the most refined metals such as silver, gold, copper, titanium, and mostly stainless steel. The most practical and popular disposable metal needle is made of stainless steel because it does not tarnish like silver or corrode like gold. For the most part, it is hypoallergenic. Titanium is better for the few patients who are hypersensitive even to stainless steel and this is an option open to the practitioner.

Nowadays it is more practical, safe and even required in some states of the United States, to use disposable needles to guard against the transmission of infectious disease. Patients are less apprehensive about treatment, and the practitioner's time is freed from sterilizing contaminated needles, which can be dangerous. The cost of disposable needles is not great and so not prohibitive. Used needles should be disposed of in biohazard containers and processed by a biohazard service for proper disposal.

■ Parts of the Needle, Lengths, and Gauges

Needle parts are important. The needle is composed of four parts—the handle, the root, the body, and the tip. The body and tip of the needle must always be sterile and never contaminated through touch or any other means, as this can contribute to the transmission of infectious disease.

An important part of the needle is the root. The root is the juncture of the handle and the body of the needle. The needle must never be inserted with less than 0.25 in of the root exposed. This allowance helps prevent a deeper penetration of the needle that might inadvertently happen if the patient moves, a muscle twitches, or the needle sinks deeper into the body due to muscle relaxation or other factors such as being touched.

Needle length is important and proper needle lengths must be selected. Most acupuncture points have a depth of insertion of 0.5 to 1.0 in, so in acupuncture practice the most common needles used are 1 in and 1.5 in. Needle length is chosen by the depth of insertion of the acupuncture point, meaning the range in which the *qi* resides in each acupuncture point. Figure 1.1 illustrates the parts of the needle and the proper depth of insertion on a 1 in needle and Table 1.**1** summarizes the most accepted depths of insertions of all the acupuncture points of the 12 main channels.

The gauge of the needle refers to the diameter or the thickness of the needle. Gauges are selected depending on the points to be treated, for in-

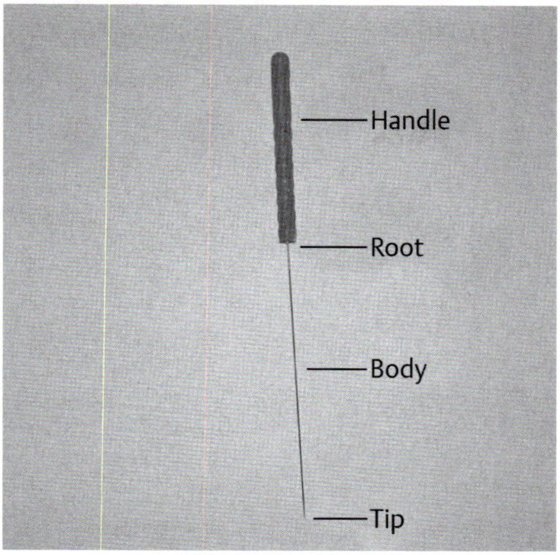

Fig. 1.1 The parts of the needle.

Channel	Depth of insertion (in)
Lung	
LU-1	0.5 – 0.8 obliquely towards the lateral aspect
LU-2	0.5 – 0.8 obliquely towards the lateral aspect
LU-3	0.5 – 1 ppd.* No moxa as a Window to the Sky point
LU-4	0.5 – 1 ppd
LU-5	0.5 – 1 ppd. No moxa, may shorten the tendon
LU-6	0.5 – 1 ppd
LU-7	0.3 – 0.5 obliquely
LU-8	0.1 – 0.3 ppd. No moxa, as the point is on the course of the radial artery
LU-9	0.2 – 0.3 Shallow insertion on course of the radial artery
LU-10	0.5 – 0.8 ppd
LU-11	0.1 or obliquely upward prick to bleed. No moxa, as it is a point to release heat
Large intestine	
LI-1	0.1 or obliquely prick to bleed
LI-2	0.2 – 0.3 ppd
LI-3	0.5 – 0.8 ppd
LI-4	0.5 – 1 ppd. **Forbidden** in Pregnancy: no moxa and needle
LI-5	0.3 – 0.5 ppd
LI-6	0.5 – 0.8 obliquely
LI-7	0.5 – 1 ppd
LI-8	0.5 – 1 ppd
LI-9	0.5 – 1 ppd
LI-10	0.8 – 1.2 ppd
LI-11	1 – 1.5 ppd
LI-12	0.5 – 1 ppd
LI-13	0.5 – 1 ppd. **Forbidden** to needle due to location on the course of the radial collateral artery and vein
LI-14	0.8 – 1.5 ppd or obliquely upward
LI-15	0.8 – 1.5 ppd or obliquely
LI-16	0.5 – 0.7 ppd
LI-17	0.3 – 0.5 ppd
LI-18	0.3 – 0.5 ppd
LI-19	0.2 – 0.3 obliquely
LI-20	0.3 – 0.5 obliquely or subcutaneously
Stomach	
ST-1	0.5 – 1 ppd. Push eye up to needle. No manipulation. No moxa
ST-2	0.2 – 0.3 ppd
ST-3	0.3 – 0.5 ppd
ST-4	1 – 1.5 subcutaneously to ST-6

* ppd = perpendicularly.

Table 1.1 Depths of insertion of the points of the 12 main channels

Channel	Depth of insertion (in)
ST-5	0.3 – 0.5 obliquely, posteriorly. Avoid the facial artery
ST-6	0.3 – 0.5 ppd or subcutaneously towards ST-4
ST-7	0.3 – 0.5 ppd
ST-8	0.5 – 1 subcutaneously
ST-9	0.3 – 0.5 ppd. **Caution** as the point is on the bifurcation of the carotid artery. No moxa
ST-10	0.3 – 0.5 ppd
ST-11	0.3 – 0.5 ppd
ST-12	0.3 – 0.5 ppd. Watch depth
ST-13	0.3 – 0.5 lateral obliquely. **Caution** as the point is over the lungs
ST-14	0.3 – 0.5 obliquely
ST-15	0.3 – 0.5 obliquely
ST-16	0.3 – 0.5 obliquely
ST-17	**Forbidden** point, the nipple, no needle, no moxa
ST-18	0.3 – 0.5 obliquely
ST-19	0.5 – 0.8 ppd. Careful of the liver
ST-20	0.5 – 1 ppd
ST-21	0.8 – 1 ppd. Careful of the liver
ST-22	0.8 – 1 ppd
ST-23	0.7 – 1 ppd
ST-24	0.7 – 1 ppd
ST-25	0.7 – 1.2 ppd
ST-26	0.7 – 1.2 ppd
ST-27	0.7 – 1.2 ppd
ST-28	0.7 – 1.2 ppd
ST-29	0.7 – 1.2 ppd
ST-30	0.5 – 1 ppd
ST-31	1 – 1.5 ppd
ST-32	1 – 1.5 ppd
ST-33	0.7 – 1 ppd
ST-34	0.5 – 1 ppd
ST-35	0.7 – 1 ppd
ST-36	0.5 – 1.2 ppd
ST-37	0.5 – 1.2 ppd
ST-38	0.5 – 1 ppd
ST-39	0.5 – 1 ppd
ST-40	0.5 – 1 ppd
ST-41	0.5 – 0.7 ppd
ST-42	0.3 – 0.5 ppd. Avoid the dorsal artery
ST-43	0.3 – 0.5 ppd
ST-44	0.3 – 0.5 ppd
ST-45	0.1 obliquely
Spleen	
SP-1	0.1 obliquely
SP-2	0.1 – 0.3 ppd
SP-3	0.3 – 0.5 ppd
SP-4	0.5 – 0.8 ppd
SP-5	0.2 – 0.3 ppd
SP-6	0.5 – 1 ppd. **Forbidden** point in pregnancy: no moxa, no needle
SP-7	0.5 – 1 ppd
SP-8	0.5 – 1 ppd
SP-9	0.5 – 1 ppd
SP-10	0.5 – 1.2 ppd
SP-11	0.5 – 1 ppd

Table 1.**1** Depths of insertion of the points of the 12 main channels (cont.)

Channel	Depth of insertion (in)
SP-12	0.5–1 ppd. Avoid the femoral artery
SP-13	0.5–1 ppd
SP-14	0.5–1 ppd
SP-15	0.7–1.2 ppd
SP-16	0.5–1 ppd
SP-17	0.3–0.5 obliquely
SP-18	0.3–0.5 obliquely
SP-19	0.3–0.5 obliquely
SP-20	0.3–0.5 obliquely
SP-21	0.3–0.5 obliquely
Heart	
HT-1	0.5–1 ppd. Avoid the axillary artery
HT-2	0.3–0.5 ppd
HT-3	0.5–1 ppd
HT-4	0.3–0.5 ppd
HT-5	0.3–0.5 ppd
HT-6	0.3–0.5 ppd
HT-7	0.3–0.5 ppd
HT-8	0.3–0.5 ppd
HT-9	0.1 subcutaneously or prick
Small intestine	
SI-1	0.1 subcutaneously or prick
SI-2	0.3–0.5 ppd
SI-3	0.5–0.7 ppd
SI-4	0.3–0.5 ppd
SI-5	0.3–0.5 ppd
SI-6	0.3–0.5 ppd
SI-7	0.5–0.8 ppd
SI-9	0.5–1 ppd

Channel	Depth of insertion (in)
SI-10	0.5–1 ppd
SI-11	0.5–1 ppd or obliquely
SI-12	0.5–0.7 ppd
SI-13	0.3–0.5 ppd
SI-14	0.3–0.7 obliquely
SI-15	0.3–0.6 obliquely
SI-16	0.3–0.7 ppd
SI-17	0.5–0.7 ppd
SI-18	0.5–0.8 ppd
SI-19	0.3–1 ppd with the mouth open
Bladder	
BL-1	0.3–0.7 ppd
BL-2	0.3–0.5 subcutaneously
BL-3	0.3–0.5 subcutaneously
BL-4	0.3–0.5 subcutaneously
BL-5	0.3–0.5 subcutaneously
BL-6	0.3–0.5 subcutaneously
BL-7	0.3–0.5 subcutaneously
BL-8	0.3–0.5 subcutaneously
BL-9	0.3–0.5 subcutaneously
BL-10	0.5–0.8 ppd
BL-11	0.5–0.7 obliquely
BL-12	0.5–0.7 obliquely
BL-13	0.5–0.7 obliquely
BL-14	0.5–0.7 obliquely
BL-15	0.5–0.7 obliquely
BL-16	0.5–0.7 obliquely
BL-17	0.5–0.7 obliquely
BL-18	0.5–0.7 obliquely

Table 1.**1** Depths of insertion of the points of the 12 main channels (cont.)

Channel	Depth of insertion (in)
BL-19	0.5 – 0.8 obliquely
BL-20	0.5 – 0.7 obliquely
BL-21	0.5 – 0.8 obliquely
BL-22	0.5 – 1 ppd
BL-23	1 – 1.2 ppd
BL-24	0.8 – 1.2 ppd
BL-25	0.8 – 1.2 ppd
BL-26	0.8 – 1.2 ppd
BL-27	0.8 – 1.2 ppd
BL-28	0.8 – 1.2 ppd
BL-29	0.8 – 1.2 ppd
BL-30	0.8 – 1.2 ppd
BL-31	0.8 – 1.2 ppd
BL-32	0.8 – 1.2 ppd
BL-33	0.8 – 1.2 ppd
BL-34	0.8 – 1.2 ppd
BL-35	0.5 – 1 ppd
BL-36	1 – 1.5 ppd
BL-37	1 – 2 ppd
BL-38	0.5 – 1 ppd
BL-39	0.5 – 1 ppd
BL-40	0.5 – 1 ppd. No moxa, may shorten the tendon
BL-41	0.3 – 0.5 ppd
BL-42	0.3 – 0.5 obliquely
BL-43	0.3 – 0.5 obliquely
BL-44	0.3 – 0.5 obliquely
BL-45	0.3 – 0.5 obliquely
BL-46	0.3 – 0.5 obliquely
BL-47	0.3 – 0.5 obliquely
BL-48	0.3 – 0.5 obliquely
BL-49	0.3 – 0.5 obliquely
BL-50	0.3 – 0.5 obliquely
BL-51	0.3 – 0.5 obliquely
BL-52	0.5 – 1 ppd
BL-53	0.8 – 1.2 ppd
BL-54	1.5 – 2 ppd
BL-55	0.7 – 1 ppd
BL-56	0.8 – 1.2 ppd
BL-57	0.8 – 1.2 ppd
BL-58	0.7 – 1 ppd
BL-59	0.5 – 1 ppd
BL-60	0.5 – 1 ppd. No needle in pregnancy
BL-61	0.3 – 0.5 ppd
BL-62	0.3 – 0.5 ppd
BL-63	0.3 – 0.5 ppd
BL-64	0.3 – 0.5 ppd
BL-65	0.3 – 0.5 ppd
BL-66	0.2 – 0.3 ppd
BL-67	0.1
Kidney	
KI-1	0.3 – 0.5 ppd
KI-2	0.3 – 0.5 ppd
KI-3	0.3 – 0.5 ppd
KI-4	0.3 – 0.5 ppd
KI-5	0.3 – 0.5 ppd
KI-6	0.3 – 0.5 ppd or horizontally posteriorly

Table 1.**1** Depths of insertion of the points of the 12 main channels (cont.)

Channel	Depth of insertion (in)
KI-7	0.5–0.7 ppd
KI-8	0.5–0.7 ppd
KI-9	0.5–0.7 ppd
KI-10	0.8–1 ppd
KI-11	0.5–1 ppd
KI-12	0.5–1 ppd
KI-13	0.5–1 ppd
KI-14	0.5–1 ppd
KI-15	0.5–1 ppd
KI-16	0.5–1 ppd
KI-17	0.5–1 ppd
KI-18	0.5–1 ppd
KI-19	0.5–1 ppd
KI-20	0.5–1 ppd
KI-21	0.3–0.7 ppd. **Caution** close to the liver
KI-22	0.3–0.5 obliquely
KI-23	0.3–0.5 obliquely
KI-24	0.3–0.5 obliquely
KI-25	0.3–0.5 obliquely
KI-26	0.3–0.5 obliquely
KI-27	0.3–0.5 obliquely
Pericardium	
PC-1	0.2–0.4 obliquely
PC-2	0.5–0.7 ppd
PC-3	0.5–0.7 ppd or bleed
PC-4	0.5–1 ppd
PC-5	0.5–1 ppd
PC-6	0.5–0.8 ppd
PC-7	0.3–0.5 ppd
PC-8	0.3–0.5 ppd
PC-9	0.1 ppd
Triple burner	
TB-1	0.1 ppd or prick
TB-2	0.3–0.5 obliquely toward the metacarpal bones
TB-3	0.3–0.5 ppd
TB-4	0.3–0.5 ppd
TB-5	0.5–1 ppd
TB-6	0.8–1.2 ppd
TB-7	0.5–1 ppd
TB-8	0.5–1 ppd. Classically **forbidden** to needle as the group *luo* of the three-arm *yang*
TB-9	0.5–1 ppd
TB-10	0.3–0.5 ppd
TB-11	0.3–0.5 ppd
TB-12	0.5–0.7 ppd
TB-13	0.5–0.8 ppd
TB-14	0.7–1 ppd
TB-15	0.3–0.5 ppd
TB-16	0.3–0.5 ppd
TB-17	0.5–1 ppd
TB-18	0.3–0.5 subcutaneously or bleed
TB-19	0.3–0.5 obliquely
TB-20	0.3–0.5 subcutaneously
TB-21	0.3–0.5 ppd with the mouth open
TB-22	0.1–0.3 obliquely
TB-23	0.3–0.5 subcutaneously. No moxa due to proximity to the eye

Table 1.**1** Depths of insertion of the points of the 12 main channels (cont.)

Channel	Depth of insertion (in)
Gall bladder	
GB-1	0.3–0.5 subcutaneously. No moxa due to proximity to the eye
GB-2	0.5–0.7 ppd
GB-3	0.3–0.5 ppd
GB-4	0.3–0.5 subcutaneously
GB-5	0.3–0.5 subcutaneously
GB-6	0.3–0.5 subcutaneously
GB-7	0.3–0.5 subcutaneously
GB-8	0.3–0.5 subcutaneously
GB-9	0.3–0.5 subcutaneously. No moxa on this point within the hairline
GB-10	0.3–0.5 subcutaneously
GB-11	0.3–0.5 subcutaneously
GB-12	0.3–0.5 obliquely
GB-13	0.3–0.5 subcutaneously
GB-14	0.3–0.5 subcutaneously
GB-15	0.3–0.5 subcutaneously
GB-16	0.3–0.5 subcutaneously
GB-17	0.3–0.5 subcutaneously
GB-18	0.3–0.5 subcutaneously
GB-19	0.3–0.5 subcutaneously
GB-20	0.5–0.8 towards the tip of the nose
GB-21	0.3–0.5 ppd
GB-22	0.3–0.5 obliquely
GB-23	0.3–0.5 obliquely
GB-24	0.3–0.5 obliquely
GB-25	0.3–0.5 ppd
GB-26	0.5–0.8 ppd
GB-27	0.5–1 ppd
GB-28	0.5–1 ppd
GB-29	0.5–1 ppd
GB-30	1.5–2.5 ppd
GB-31	0.7–1.2 ppd
GB-32	0.7–1 ppd
GB-33	0.5–1 ppd
GB-34	0.8–1.2 ppd
GB-35	0.5–0.8 ppd
GB-36	0.5–0.8 ppd
GB-37	0.7–1 ppd
GB-38	0.5–0.7 ppd
GB-39	0.3–0.5 ppd
GB-40	0.5–0.8 ppd
GB-41	0.3–0.5 ppd
GB-42	0.3–0.5 ppd. No moxa due to dorsal artery and venous network
GB-43	0.3–0.5 ppd
GB-44	0.1 subcutaneously
Liver	
LR-1	0.1–0.2 obliquely
LR-2	0.3–0.5 obliquely
LR-3	0.3–0.5 ppd
LR-4	0.3–0.5 ppd
LR-5	0.3–0.5 subcutaneously posteriorly horizontally
LR-6	0.5–0.8 subcutaneously horizontally
LR-7	0.5–1 ppd (0.4–0.6 range)
LR-8	0.5–0.8 ppd
LR-9	0.5–0.7 ppd
LR-10	0.5–1 ppd

Table 1.**1** Depths of insertion of the points of the 12 main channels (cont.)

Channel	Depth of insertion (in)
LR-11	0.5–1 ppd
LR-12	Moxa, no needle due to the femoral artery and vein
LR-13	0.5–0.8 ppd. Moxa three to five minutes
LR-14	0.5–0.8 obliquely towards the lateral aspect
Conception vessel	
CV-1	0.5–1 ppd
CV-2	0.5–1 ppd
CV-3	0.5–1 ppd
CV-4	0.8–1.2 ppd
CV-5	0.5–1 ppd
CV-6	0.8–1.2 ppd
CV-7	0.8–1.2 ppd
CV-8	Umbilicus, **forbidden** to needle, moxa fine
CV-9	0.5–1 ppd
CV-10	0.5–1.2 ppd
CV-11	0.5–1.2 ppd
CV-12	0.5–1.2 ppd
CV-13	0.5–1.2 ppd
CV-14	0.3–0.8 ppd
CV-15	0.4–0.6 obliquely or horizontally
CV-16	0.3–0.5 subcutaneously
CV-17	0.3–0.5 subcutaneously upwards
CV-18	0.3–0.5 subcutaneously
CV-19	0.3–0.5 subcutaneously
CV-20	0.3–0.5 subcutaneously
CV-21	0.3–0.5 subcutaneously

Channel	Depth of insertion (in)
CV-22	0.2 subcutaneously (then 0.5–1 downward)
CV-23	0.2–0.3 obliquely upward towards the tongue root
CV-24	0.2–0.3 obliquely upward
Governing vessel	
GV-1	0.5–1 ppd
GV-2	0.5–1 obliquely upward
GV-3	0.5–1 ppd
GV-4	0.5–1 ppd
GV-5	0.5–1 ppd
GV-6	0.5–1 ppd. No moxa, may move the spine
GV-7	0.5–1 ppd. No moxa, may move the spine
GV-8	0.5–1 ppd
GV-9	0.5–1 obliquely upward
GV-10	0.5–1 obliquely. Classically **forbidden** to needle due to connection with the heart
GV-11	0.5–1 obliquely upward
GV-12	0.5–1 obliquely upward
GV-13	0.5–1 obliquely upward
GV-14	0.5–1 obliquely upward
GV-15	0.5–0.8 ppd. No moxa on this point at the nape
GV-16	0.5–0.8 ppd, not deep. No moxa, as a Window to the Sky point
GV-17	0.3–0.5 subcutaneously
GV-18	0.3–0.5 subcutaneously
GV-19	0.3–0.5 subcutaneously
GV-20	0.3–0.5 subcutaneously

Table 1.**1** Depths of insertion of the points of the 12 main channels (cont.)

Channel	Depth of insertion (in)
GV-21	0.3 – 0.5 subcutaneously
GV-22	0.3 – 0.5 subcutaneously
GV-23	0.3 – 0.5 subcutaneously or bleed
GV-24	0.3 – 0.5 subcutaneously or bleed
GV-25	0.2 – 0.3 ppd or bleed. No moxa, due to proximity to nose and connection to brain
GV-26	0.3 – 0.5 obliquely upward. No moxa, due to proximity to nose and connection to brain
GV-27	0.2 – 0.3 ppd
GV-28	0.1 – 0.2 obliquely upward or bleed

Table 1.**1** Depths of insertion of the points of the 12 main channels (cont.)

stance, the texture of the skin they are located on. For thick skin such as the scalp or the ear, use a thick needle such as a 28 g (gauge) or 30 g. When needling the delicate skin of the face, use a thin needle such as a 36 g.

Careful attention to needle length and gauge helps to achieve the desired therapeutic result. See the next section below for a summary of the selection criteria for needle length and gauge (see also Fig. 1.**2**) and a conversion table of Chinese and Japanese needle measurements (Table 1.**2**), as Chinese and Japanese measurement systems are different.

Selecting a Needle

When selecting a needle to treat a particular acupuncture point there are always two parameters to consider:

- The depth of insertion of the *qi* of the channel suggests the length of the needle.
- The tissues to be needled, such as delicate face points or thick muscles or cartilage, require thin or thicker gauge or thicker needles respectively. For example, a shallow face point would be needled best with a short, thin needle, and a deep muscular point should be needled with a long, relatively thicker needle.

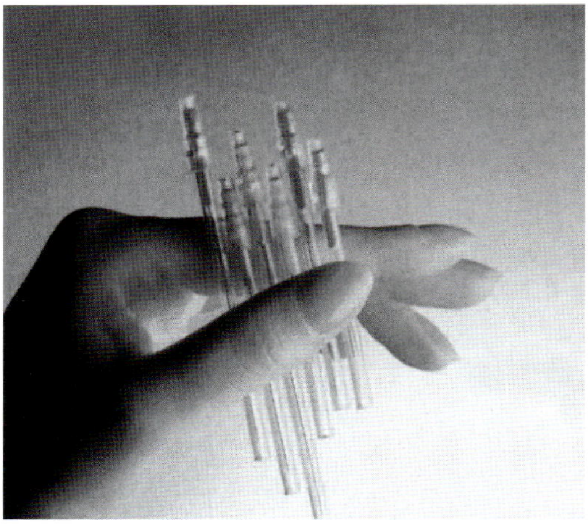

Fig. 1.**2** Needles come in various lengths and gauges. Courtesy of Seirin Europe/3B Scientific, Hamburg, Germany.

Gauge (Thickness)

The thickness or diameter of the needle is called the gauge (g). The most common Chinese needle gauges are 28 g, 30 g, 32 g, 34 g, and 36 g. The bigger the number, the smaller the gauge or thickness. For example, a 28 g needle is much thicker than a 36 g. Often, 28 g needles are used in the ear, on *jing* (well) points to bleed, and on the scalp. The most common needles used on the body are 34 g.

The most common Japanese needles are #1, #3, and #5 gauges. In the Japanese system, the bigger the number, the bigger the gauge or thickness. A #1 needle is thin and a #5 is thick. A #5 is used in the ear and on *jing* (well) points. A #1 is very fine (and my favorite). A #3 is used on body points along with #1 needles. For practitioner convenience other gauges are listed in Table 1.**2**.

Length

The length of the needle is measured in millimeters or inches. Select needle length according to the depth of insertion and in consideration of the patient's body:

- 15 mm = 0.5 in—use for ear, and *jing* (well) points;
- 30 mm = 1 in—use for average depth body points;

Japanese Gauges	#00	#01	#1	#2	#3	#5	#8
mm	0.12	0.14	0.16	0.18	0.20	0.25	0.30
Seirin J-Type needles (Japanese); color code of the handle	dark green	lime green	red	ivory	blue	blue	brown
Chinese equivalent			36 g		34 g	30 g	

Table 1.**2** Japanese needle gauges and lengths and their equivalents in different systems

- 40 mm = 1.5 in—use for patients who have more muscle or adipose tissue or on points with deeper depths of insertion.

See below for options in common needle lengths:

- 30 mm = 1 in;
- 40 mm = 1.5 in;
- 50 mm = 2 in.

Angle of Insertion

The angle of insertion, or how to position the needle, is also another important needle parameter. Most acupuncture points, because of their location, can simply be needled by a perpendicular insertion. A small percentage of points need to be inserted obliquely or transversely because of the proximity to organs, arteries, or other delicate structures. If a point is needled obliquely, consider the direction of the oblique insertion as well, that is, which way that oblique insertion is positioned.

Even points that are normally inserted perpendicularly can be needled obliquely if you are using the angle of insertion as either a tonification or a dispersion technique. In this case, needle the point in the direction of the channel, which means in the direction of the *qi* flow. For instance, with Lung 7 (*lie que*), angle the needle distally towards LU-9 (*tai yuan*) to tonify. To disperse the point, needle the point proximally against the flow of the channel, that is, from LU-7 (*lie que*) to LU-5 (*chi ze*).

Luo points, a special category of points that either connect to the source point of the coupled organ (i. e., Lung 7 to Large Intestine 4), or stimulate the pertaining organ, i. e., the lung, may be needled according to the trajectory of the channel without necessarily tonifying or dispersing. This difference in use is achieved by the actual, physical angle of insertion. For an extensive discussion of *luo* points see my first textbook *Holding the Tiger's Tail.*[1]

Angles of insertion are important. Overall, you should have a good sense of them through study and by looking at the person's body. If need be, you can always look them up for accuracy and safety, but careful attention to observation and feeling, along with study, should serve you well.

Patient Positioning

Most practitioners know that proper patient positioning for needling is essential. Patients may be positioned reclining on their stomach, back, sometimes on their side, or seated, again depending upon the points to be treated. Make sure the neck always receives proper support and is not turned too far in either direction or kept for too long in any one position.

Sometimes the patient may be seated for needling as in the case of bleeding a *jing* (well) point on the foot or hand, or seated with their head forward and resting on a pillow to access points like Gall Bladder 20 (*feng chi*) or others at the nape. All points need to be accessible so it is a good idea for patients to wear a gown for needling points on the torso, back, or upper legs and arms. Changing out of street clothes also assists the patient in the transition from their normal state to one of healing and relaxation. Always automatically drape the patient carefully to promote modesty.

Be sure to provide the patient with as much comfort as possible by setting up the treatment table in advance with a comfortable pillow, a table covering such as a disposable sheet over a blanket, a bolster for their knees if needed, and a disposable drape sheet to cover them directly, along with a lightweight fleece blanket on top if temperatures demand. Keep the feet covered to retain body temperature.

Before needling, make contact with the patient's body by palpating the points that have been selected to needle. Scan the skin for surface tension and temperature with your hand, and gently press the points to be needled perpendicularly to assess tension, hardness, lumps or softness. A general rule of thumb is never to needle into tense, hard tissue, so if you feel this select a more distal, related point to needle.

Needling tense, tight tissue causes discomfort to the patient, but also increases the difficulty of needling to the proper depth, inhibits *qi* arrival, may cause unnecessary pain upon insertion, or bend or break the needle. Various massage and palpatory skills as well as the application of moxa or the TDP lamp (a therapeutic infrared device) may assist in loosening tight tissue before needle insertion. Additionally, palpation helps both in bringing *qi* to the area if need be, or in dispersing it if it is stagnant, and actually transforms the tissues, making them more energetically active. Palpation also prepares the patient mentally and physically for needling. The needle can be properly inserted once surface tension is relieved.

The Insertion Tube

The method of needle insertion is one of practitioner preference, and either style—freehanded or with an insertion tube—are options. Many patients prefer the gentleness of the Japanese needle with an insertion tube because of the overall superior manufactured quality of the needle and the benefits of using the tube, but regardless of which method is selected, needle insertion should always be painless.

A Japanese needle with the insertion tube is an easy painless way to insert a needle both gently and sterilely, such that the force of insertion sometimes caused by a freehanded insertion does not overcome the patient. The insertion tube has several functions that contribute to its usefulness and it can be helpful to review them as well as how to use this type of needle properly:

- The insertion tube assists in a perpendicular, oblique, or transverse insertion. The practitioner simply needs to hold the needle at whatever angle is desired for insertion—perpendicular, oblique, or transverse—and then hits the needle as discussed below.
- Correct use of an insertion tube requires two hands. Some practitioners awkwardly use only one hand when attempting to insert a needle with an insertion tube. They hold the tube with one hand and then simultaneously try to hit the needle with the same hand. This is incorrect. Done this way the practitioner lacks the force to hit the handle of the needle because his/her fingers are spread out in too many directions doing too many things, and that lack of strength means the needle is not hit firmly enough to pierce the skin. To use the insertion tube correctly, hold the insertion tube with your left hand and hit the handle of the needle that is extending beyond the tube with a firm, quick, tap with your right index finger if you are right-handed. Do the opposite if you are left-handed. Using two hands gives you more control over the needle and the force to hit the needle into the skin.
- The insertion tube spreads the free nerve endings, which promotes painless insertion. Always disengage the needle from the tube before touching the point so you don't exert more pressure and cause pain by disengaging the needle with the needle tip on the skin. Put the insertion tube down on the point to be needled and press down slightly on the tube so when you hit the handle of the needle that extends beyond the tube it will go in because you have already made an indentation for it. Tell the patient that what they are feeling is the tube, which is spreading the free nerve endings at its base. Without hesitation, quickly hit the needle handle so that it pierces the skin. Some practitioners repeatedly hit the part of the handle that is sticking above the tube in a series of small taps. Most patients report that this is annoying and even painful as the tip is inserted slowly and repeatedly. One firm tap fulfills one of the functions of the insertion tube—painless penetration through the free nerve endings. Once the tube is positioned properly, immediately push the needle to the depth at which *qi* resides (the standard depth of insertion). Complete the needling process by getting *qi* and then by manipulating the *qi* with either a tonification or dispersion technique.

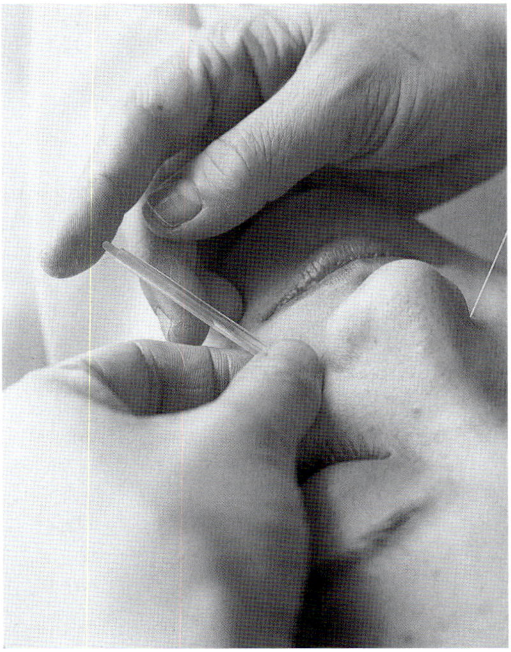

Fig. 1.3 The insertion tube. Courtesy of Seirin Europe/3B Scientific, Hamburg, Germany.

- The insertion tube helps with sterile needle insertion. As a sheath, the insertion tube protects the needle from being touched and thereby contaminated.

Clean Field

All needling should be accomplished from a 'clean field.' The clean field consists of a medium-size sheet of professional toweling with all supplies laid out on it. An open alcohol jar and an open cotton ball jar may remain 'off the field' as of course can the biohazard unit. Needles, tweezers, and other implements are kept on the field.

Bent, Broken, or Stuck Needles

If the advice with regard to proper needle insertion, preparing the skin, and properly using the insertion tube is followed, the chance of broken and stuck needles is virtually non-existent. However, bent needles can occur if the practitioner uses a needle that is too thin or uses force in needle insertion.

Needle Shock and Managing Accidents

The best way to manage needle shock and acupuncture accidents (lightheadedness, faintness, for example) is to avoid them through proper needling and by paying attention to the patient's condition. However, some precautions and emergency procedures are summarized below:

- Do not treat patients who are too weak, too tired or too hungry.
- Do not treat patients who have eaten too much, are intoxicated or on mind-altering drugs.
- Correctly position the patient for needling.
- Do not needle too forcefully, too deeply, for too long, or with too many needles.
- If signs of needle shock/acupuncture sickness develop, stay calm, withdraw all needles, elevate the feet, cover the torso with a blanket, and press on resuscitation points such as GV-26 (*ren zhong*) or KI-1 (*yong quan*), and administer a warm drink when conscious. GV-26 will bring the energy up to the head if the patient is dizzy or lightheaded, and KI-1 will bring the energy down if the person is nervous or needs to be grounded. Signs of acupuncture sickness include the following:
  - pallor;
  - shallow or rapid breathing;
  - unconsciousness or fainting;
  - sweaty hands, face, chest, or feet;
  - lightheadedness;
  - increased or decreased body temperature.

If the patient is unconscious, which is a serious matter, determine a carotid pulse, call an emergency phone number, administer CPR if needed, and then perform the above procedures.

Now that the foundation has been laid for treatment we can proceed to discuss the next layer of needle techniques.

Reference

1. Gardner-Abbate S. *Holding the Tiger's Tail: An Acupuncture Techniques Manual in the Treatment of Disease*. Santa Fe: Southwest Acupuncture College Press; 1996.

2 Thoughts on Needling within the Clinical Encounter

Before engaging in a discussion on needle techniques and protocols, let us first look at what could be called a general treatment framework on the art of needling and where it fits into the clinical schema. Thoughts and tips are offered to the practitioner to illustrate the infrastructure of the treatment setting and the elegant simplicity of treating within the Oriental medical model.

In 1988, I embarked on my first trip to China with the express purpose of improving my needle technique. When I analyzed my abilities at that time after 5 years of clinical practice, I found that diagnosis and treatment plans were easy for me but that my needle technique was less than adequate. For the most part, my patients returned for treatment and got better, but I was tentative with needling and the administration of the treatment. I was an acupuncturist who was nervous and uncomfortable with acupuncture!

Like the experiences of most practitioners who have traveled to China, it is not surprising that there I witnessed a strong needling style by the Chinese doctors I studied with. Large-gauge needles, a *de qi* sensation that would bring patients to tears, vigorous tonification and dispersion methods, and a general needle retention time of about 20 minutes, regardless of the condition being treated, were typical.

For six weeks I was taught in Beijing how to practice that form of acupuncture on patients who I couldn't communicate with except in rudimentary Chinese modified by my strong New England accent. Daily I'd ask, "Do you have *qi*?" or "Do you feel pain?" or more likely, "Do you feel *soup*?" since the word for pain (*tong*) I'm sure sounded more like soup (*tang*) when I said it. No wonder they looked at me askance, shaking their heads in distrust and disbelief. Nevertheless, perhaps it was because of such cultural barriers that I was uninhibited enough to develop a strong Chinese needle technique in contrast to the one I had before going to China, which was to hit the handle extending from the insertion tube, turn away from the patient, and emit a sickly scream!

Of course, there were many styles of acupuncture to observe in China and they were modified by the presentation of the patient as well as the practitioner. I fondly recall the case of an elderly gentleman who had recently had a heart attack. When he came in for treatment, the doctor positioned the man on his stomach, and with a quick in-and-out needle technique, needled Bladder 15 (*xin shu*), back *shu* point of the heart. A colleague commented that this different needling style and lack of needle retention must have been done in consideration of the patient's serious condition so as not to drain his heart *qi*.

Suspicious of this observation, before writing it down as truth in my little pocket notebook, I asked the doctor if this is what he was doing. Instantly, everyone in the room started laughing at our naive conclusion, and the doctor stated matter of factly that this was not the reason for the lack of needle retention. Rather, he had chosen this type of treatment because the patient had to leave the hospital early to catch the bus!

The first day upon my return from China as we were catching up on things, my husband told me that he had injured his back while I was away and he had resigned himself to accepting its residual pain since he had tried many therapies with limited success. Deftly, I pulled out a 30 gauge Chinese Huato needle, stuck it into Small Intestine 6 (*yang lou*) in the direction of the channel (proximally up the arm), and twirled it dispassionately and painlessly, but evoking so much *qi* that his consciousness was literally altered and his pain completely disappeared. He then said to me, "You *did* learn how to needle in China!" I now appreciated everything about acupuncture that made it effective—the length and gauge of the needle, the angle and depth of insertion needed for effective treatment, the proper *de qi* sensation—in short, the power I knew it possessed if properly engaged.

That same week I had the opportunity to study with a Japanese scholar visiting the college where I was Dean. During those few days, the exact antitheses of Chinese needling methods were demonstrated. The thinnest #1 (36 gauge) Japanese

Seirin needles were the needles of choice. They were only superficially inserted 0.1 – 0.5 in on average, usually obliquely or transversely, and no *qi* was solicited. Points were tonified or dispersed by angling the needle in relation to the direction of the channel flow versus other manual methods. Patients were hardly aware of the presence of the needles and most of them preferred this style of treatment, finding it painless and pleasant. Clinical results were immediate and efficacious.

Witnessing such dichotomous styles of treatment back to back was a turning point in my acupuncture career. Both Chinese and Japanese styles were opposite in execution and feel, but each was grounded in the same ancient theory of contacting the *qi*. In the Chinese case, needling was for the most part perpendicular and deep so that the *qi* of the channels could be contacted. In the Japanese system, needling was superficial and thereby transverse or oblique, contacting the superficial *qi* of the minute, blood and *luo* vessels (small capillary-like vessels that arise off the main channels and bring *qi* and blood to every part of the body at the level of the skin). This 180° gamut represented the range of needle options one could select from for a wide range of disorders and patient types and they have served me well. Four technique books, including this one, grew out of my clinical experience with both approaches and I am grateful for those educational opportunities that prepared me to teach and write about needle technique and to treat patients.

In reviewing my educational odyssey, a few basic ideas come to mind concerning needling, and for me they constitute the infrastructure of my treatment approach. These ideas are discussed below as tips for the student and practitioner:

1. First, my basic contention is not to make a treatment more complex than it needs to be. One way to do this is not to needle too many points on patients (especially Americans, who already have a bias against needles no matter how small because of their fear of pain from experience with childhood immunizations or other inoculations). Too many needles not only cause discomfort to the patient, and discourage them from returning, but more importantly may not target the patient's major complaint precisely enough.
2. Diagnostically, when the practitioner prioritizes the patient's symptoms over the root of the problem he/she usually selects too many points to treat. Even with a painless insertion, too many needles scatter the therapeutic intent of the treatment and disrupt the patient's equilibrium. It is understandable that when we begin to treat a patient for the first time we may feel that there are so many things we need to address that we don't know where to begin. At the risk of oversimplification, to correct this dilemma, I advise the following:
   - With regard to actual treatment, I believe that it is better to proceed slowly than with too much vigor so that the patient's response can be properly evaluated.
   - Establish a clear, concise diagnosis. The treatment plan will then follow from this and should be as apparent and succinct as the diagnosis. For example, if the patient's diagnosis is spleen *qi* vacuity, the concomitant treatment plan is to tonify the *qi* of the spleen.
   - Unless emergency treatments are administered, in which case there is the need to treat life-threatening manifestations (symptoms), the diagnosis should address the root, which is usually not multifaceted and therefore does not need many needles. By logical extension, when the root is treated it will also address its manifestations.
   - Choose points with multiple, powerful energetics to assist in an economy of points to be needled.
   - Do not be repetitive with point energetic use. Choose points based upon their unique energetics. Additional points can be selected to reinforce the treatment but repetition leads to the use of too many points.
   - Use the best quality needles available for acupuncture (in my opinion, Seirin needles). A quality needle can do wonders in making up for a less than perfect needle technique and enhances patient tolerance and satisfaction with the treatment. If you employ a needling style such as a Chinese one where you solicit *qi*, it can still be obtained with the finest of needles. If you prefer a Japanese technique where, for example, *qi* is contacted superficially via the minute *luo* vessels, and tonification and dispersion is

achieved by needle insertion with or against the direction of the flow of the channel, these needles are ideal for such shallow insertions.

The cumulative effect of this system of needling is multifold:

1. A few points are needled as painlessly as possible. Patients like this.
2. The root is treated through the clarity of the diagnosis and the points selected. This increases therapeutic effectiveness.
3. Correspondingly, treating the root generally decreases the length and course of treatment. This saves the patient time and money.
4. Patients are more likely to continue with therapy because the needling is not uncomfortable, they are experiencing improvement, and they can afford the treatment.
5. Competing signals are not given to the body by too many needles about what needs to be corrected. Clinical experience with many therapies demonstrates that, the body in its response to stimuli does not react to multiple stimuli but reacts economically by prioritizing the most threatening or larger stimulus. So, let the body know what you are trying to achieve in the treatment plan by prioritizing the points to be needled.
6. Additionally, regardless of the needle technique and point selection, the quality of the practitioner/patient relationship and their mutual trust and respect is perhaps the most important variable in patient comfort, care, and cure. While this will be discussed in my next book, *The Spiritual Practice of Clinical Medicine*, for now let me simply recommend—be yourself, be in touch with values that affirm life from conception to natural death, be truthful as you guide your patient back to balance, and be kind and compassionate.

Looking at this strategy in relation to the classics, the brilliant scholars Paul Larre and Elisabeth Rochat de la Vallee agree. They wisely point out:

> The *Huang Di Nei Jing* tells us that the healing process is not just mechanical—it is not simply the placing of a needle. The most important thing for healing is the relationship between the practitioner, the spirits, and the patient. The relationship begins with the personal attitude and inner behavior of the practitioner. Your own spirits and forces must be in good concentration in order to be able to evaluate the patient and to be able to rectify what is wrong in the movement of his or her vitality. It is your spirit which enables you to make the diagnosis, choose the points, and give a feeling of rightness to the patient at a high level—without interfering with the patient's freedom. The treatment always takes place inside of this practitioner–patient relationship.[1]

Let us keep these general treatment strategies in mind as we explore advanced techniques for the treatment of disease in Oriental medicine.

Reference

1. Larre P, Rochat de la Vallee E. The practitioner–patient relationship. *J Trad Acu*. Winter 1990 – 91: 14 – 17 and 48 – 50.

3 Treating the Spirit—Treating the Blood with Oriental Medicine

Physicians of old have recognized the importance of tending the spirit in order to treat disease effectively. In particular, the *Huang Di Nei Jing* (*Yellow Emperor's Classic of Medicine*), the oldest extant Chinese medical text (500 – 300 BC), states that in order to treat illness one must first establish contact with the patient's spirit. This is certainly easier to do with a paradigm such as Oriental medicine, which sees no separation between the body, mind, and spirit, since they are viewed as inextricable components of the life force. However, the classical exhortation reminds us that the spirit is the motive force of the organism and must be reached first in order to initiate the healing process.

In Oriental medicine, the acupuncture needle is often seen as the instrument of contacting the spirit because the needles are inserted into discrete acupuncture points, each of which is said to control specific physiological functions of the body down to the cellular level—indeed, what we might think of as the innate wisdom or spirit of the body. Correspondingly, acupuncture points are named according to that spirit, but Oriental medicine also recognizes that before a practitioner can physically stick a needle into someone, another form of "spirit connecting" beyond the cellular level is essential as well. As most successful practitioners acknowledge, whether it is through guided imagery, eye contact, laughter, a smile, a handshake, or the ability to listen and be present for the patient, satisfying medicine for both the practitioner and the patient requires meaningful interaction—a deeper, soulful, spiritual encounter. The three treasures diagnostic paradigm reminds us that, of the three treasures—*jing*, *qi*, and *shen*—*shen* (spirit) must be treated first. It must be balanced, rooted, and secured before the manipulation of *qi* for it is indeed our core substrate, the motive force of the body and mind.

There are several ways to treat the spirit through needling acupuncture points with specific energetics. One particular approach that I have incorporated follows the ancient tenet that "Blood is the material basis of the human spirit." The blood is the basis of our essence and of our mental and emotional activities. Thus, by regulating the blood, the spirit can be tangibly addressed.

Most acupuncture points treat the blood or the *qi* as the material basis of the *yin* and the *yang*. For ease of understanding and use, the following five points are amongst my favorite acupuncture points to treat the spirit by treating the blood. Their locations, energetics, and the specific needle techniques that can be used are discussed below.

■ PC-6 *Nei Guan* (Inner Gate)

Location

Standard Chinese location. PC-6 can be found 2 *cun* above the transverse crease of the wrist between the tendons of the palmaris longus and flexor carpi radialis muscles.

Energetics

My favorite point in treating the blood is *nei guan*, PC-6. Pericardium 6 is the major point to move stagnant *qi* anywhere in the body, particularly in the upper burner. As such, it has the ability to decongest stagnant liver *qi* and to move the *qi* of the upper burner, thereby expanding the diaphragm, broadening the chest, and draining off excess stuck energy of the upper burner including stagnant emotional energy. Because the blood follows the *qi*, this point likewise moves the blood.

As a longitudinal *luo* point, Pericardium 6 regulates the *qi* and blood of the heart, opens the heart orifice, calms the spirit and the mind, and benefits the brain, the emotions, and the mental state.

Method

Puncture the point perpendicularly 0.5 to 1.0 in, or apply deep dispersive pressure to the point several times a day as needed. When using PC-6 as a longitudinal *luo*, needle the point obliquely 0.3 to 0.5 in in the distal direction (towards the fingers). Magnetic wrist bracelets (for sea sickness) worn on the point perform these functions well.

■ KI-6 *Zhao Hai* (Shining Sea)

Location

My preferred location of KI-6 is what is typically referred to as Japanese KI-6 (which is actually one of the alternative Chinese locations). This location is defined as 1 *cun* directly below the medial malleolus at the junction of the red and the white skin.

Energetics

KI-6 is my second favorite point of choice for assisting the spirit by treating the blood. Kidney 6 is perhaps to Japanese acupuncture what ST-36 (*zu san li*) is to Chinese acupuncture. It is the primary point to nourish the *yin*, a vital component of the blood. By nourishing *yin*, it calms the mind, cools the blood, strengthens the adrenal glands, and supports the sympathetic nervous system. It is useful for chronic illness, stress, and trauma, which typically have an emotional (spirit) component.

Method

Puncture the point with a #1 (or 36 gauge) 30 mm needle transversely toward the heel, inserting it 0.1 to 0.2 in. Do not obtain *qi* on the point; simply insert it toward the heel. This is considered a tonification technique as it is inserted in the direction of the channel. See Figure 3.**1a** and **b** for illustration.

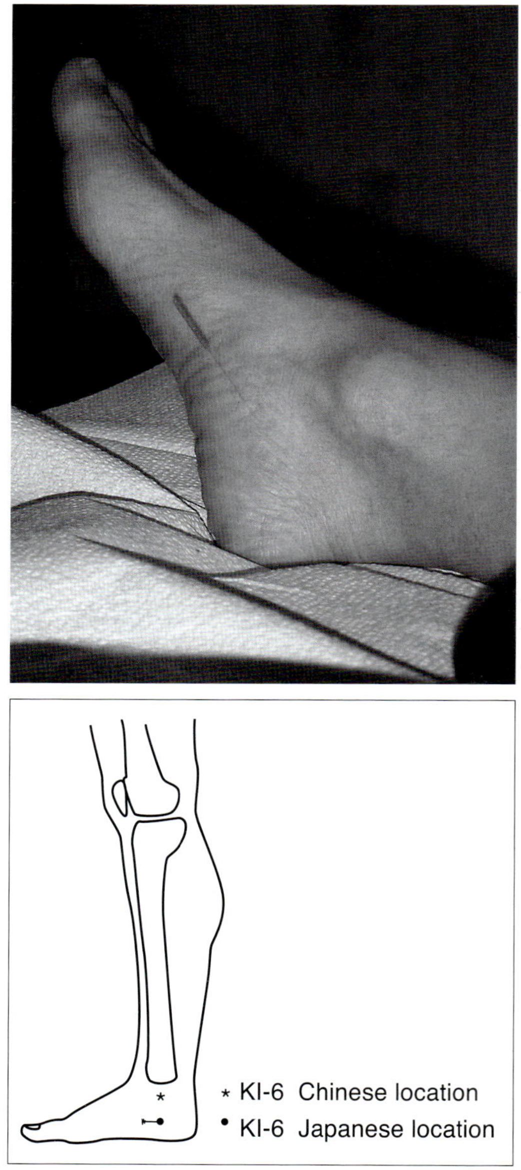

Fig. 3.**1a, b** Location and needle method for Japanese KI-6 (*zhao hai*).

■ KI-1 *Yong Quan* (Gushing Spring)

Location

Standard Chinese location—in the depression on the sole of the foot, at the junction of the upper and middle two-thirds of the sole.

Energetics

Kidney 1 is one of the most powerful points to treat the spirit and the blood. Physiologically it is the *jing* (well) point, wood point, and sedation point of the kidney channel. It tonifies *yin*, clears heat, subdues wind, calms the mind, restores consciousness, nourishes the kidney, and suppresses liver fire. In Japanese acupuncture, it is the primary point to adjust and treat any vascular disturbance such as blood stagnation, blood pressure problems, or any other circulatory problems. Many health problems, both physical and emotional, can be resolved when treating this point, due to its intimate connection to the blood.

Method

Palpate the point first to optimize its energetics. This point is extremely tender on most patients. Patients can be taught how to massage the point daily for several minutes in order to treat themselves. To consolidate the effect, the practitioner should needle it. Use a #1 or 36 gauge needle with an insertion tube to assist in inserting the needle painlessly. Puncture perpendicularly 0.3 – 0.5 in.

■ HT-7 *Shen Men* (Spirit Gate)

Location

The point may be located according to the standard Chinese location, which is on the transverse crease of the wrist, in the articular regions of the pisiform and the ulna, in the depression on the radial side of the tendon of the flexor carpi ulnaris muscle. Or it may be found alternatively in the Japanese location, which is on the medial side of the flexor carpi ulnaris tendon. In this case, the needle is simply inserted underneath the tendon of the flexor carpi ulnaris muscle towards the Chinese HT-7.

Energetics

Heart 7 (HT-7) is a primary point for treating the spirit. As the *shu* (stream) point, source point, earth point, and sedation point on the heart channel, it quiets the heart and calms the spirit. By virtue of these effects, as the classics say, "When the Heart is serene, all pain is negligible." It is a primary point for pain, emotional problems, anxiety, and insomnia. Heart 7 and Kidney 6 work synergistically to coordinate the strong relationship between the heart and the kidney, fire and water, the blood and the spirit.

Method

Puncture the Chinese point location perpendicularly 0.3 to 0.5 in or thread transversely under the tendon in the Japanese location. Obtain little or no *qi* depending on your style of treatment. The Japanese location and needle method is a handy technique when it is difficult to needle the bony Chinese location, as sometimes the patient has arthritic bone deformities or tight tendons in the area. See Figure 3.**2** for the Japanese needling method and point location.

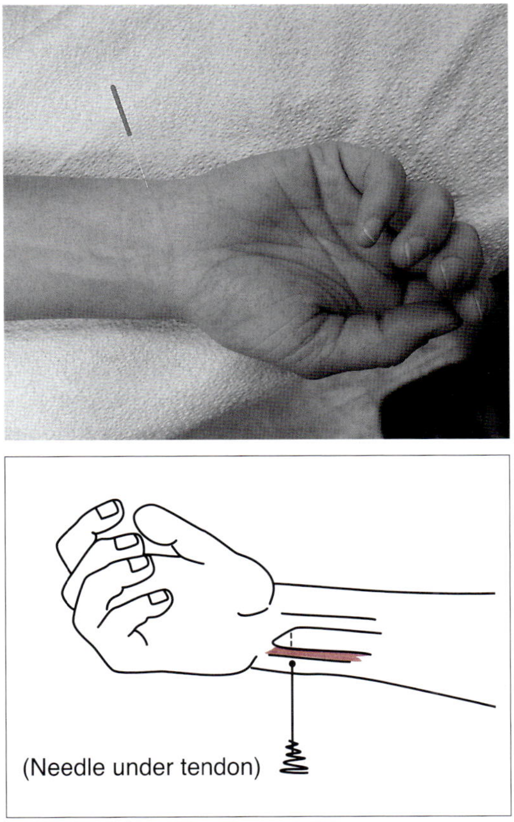

Fig. 3.**2a, b** Location and Japanese needle method for HT-7 (*shen men*).

■ SP-10 *Xue Hai* (Sea of Blood)

Location

The Chinese location of this point is defined as 2 *cun* above the medio-superior border of the patella, on the bulge of the medial portion of the quadriceps femoris muscle, when the knee is flexed. Generally, this point is extremely tender when palpated, especially in the Japanese location of the point. For this location, cup your right palm to the patient's left knee with the thumb on its medial side and the other four fingers directed proximally. The Japanese point location is where the tip of your thumb rests. It is a big area, more medial than the Chinese location. Both points are depicted in Figure 3.**3**.

Energetics

Energetically, SP-10 is a Sea of Blood point, meaning it has a profound influence on the blood. It is also a point of intersection of the *chong* channel, the extraordinary vessel that is also a reservoir of blood. Diagnostically, via palpation, it is indicative of blood stagnation anywhere in the body. It cools heat in the blood, moves, tonifies, and strengthens it. It perfuses the lower abdomen as well as activates blood.

Method

The point may be punctured bilaterally 0.7 to 1.2 in.

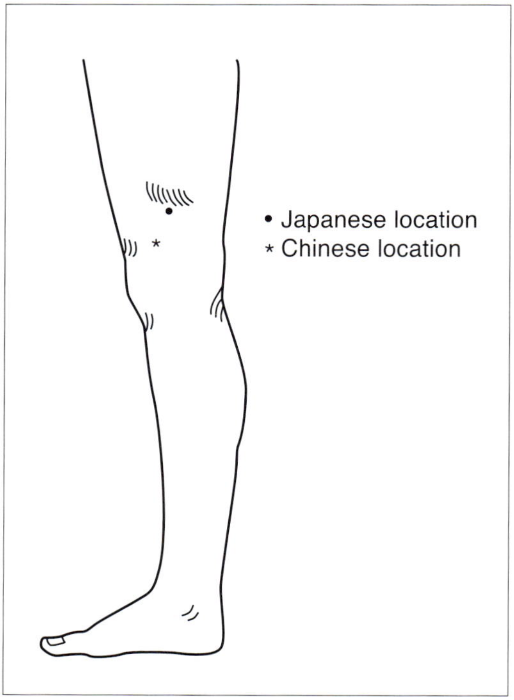

Fig. 3.**3** Two locations of SP-10 (*xue hai*).

While there are certainly other points that can be used to treat the spirit, in terms of their strong connection to the blood, these five points are extraordinarily effective. The selected use of these points as a core part of your acupuncture prescription can help you treat the spirit by treating the blood. This is surely a strength of the Oriental medical paradigm.

II The Treatment of Specific Diseases

4 Gentle Treatment for General Anxiety Disorder, Post-traumatic Stress, and Episodic Anxiety

As the *Ling Shu*, the second part of the *Huang Di Nei Jing* classic text, so wisely stated centuries ago:

> To every needling, the method is above all not to miss the rooting in the Spirits. To be effective and at the same time not to violate the organism goes all the way to the origin of the patient's life, to the place where the Spirits are rooted. The Spirits, vacillating under the emotional shock of apprehension and worry, are no longer guarded in their place and can no longer guarantee the person. There is a dispossession of that which makes the person; one loses possession of oneself.[1]

These ancient and astute words certainly speak to our times, not just for the 10 million Americans, and countless others worldwide, who on a daily basis suffer from generalized anxiety disorder (GAD—a sustained acute disorder defined as lasting 6 months or longer). Likewise, the millions who experience post-traumatic stress (defined as symptoms persisting for longer than a month after a traumatic or catastrophic event), and episodic anxiety (anxiety linked to an extraordinary life event). Such anxiety and stress can be overwhelming to the person and can manifest as social isolation, uncontrollable worry, tension, irritability, fatigue, muscular aches and pains, sleep disorders, restlessness, extreme anxiety, numbness to the event, palpitations, and startling easily.

While each of these varieties of anxiety differ in terms of their definitions, they have more in common than not. Western treatments tend to center around prescription drug therapy to assist in restoring chemical balance to the brain. Most of these drugs are designed for short-term use; some can become addictive such as the benzodiazepines like Valium and Ativan. Many produce other undesirable side-effects such as decreased appetite, dry mouth, sweating, constipation, tremor, fatigue, and sexual difficulties.

Dr. Allen Keller, a primary care physician at New York's Bellevue Hospital who heads up a group, Survivors of Torture, recommends the following mechanisms as ways to cope with anxiety and stress. As Oriental medical practitioners, we can apply these principles as well:

1. Encourage the patient to maintain social connections in the wake of their problems.
2. Don't *force* the patient to talk about the traumatic event that is affecting them. (The key word here is *force—my italics.)* However, allow them to talk about it even if all you can do is listen. You do not have to have a solution, just a compassionate ear.
3. *Acknowledge* the person's experience of the event and support them in their experience rather than emphasize the medicalization (somatizing) of their condition, that is, materializing the symptoms.
4. However, periodically check in with the person on the somatic symptoms of their distress.

This is not to say that the experience of anxiety is not real or that the somatized symptoms are false, for they are very real physically and can interfere with the person's functioning and their health. Our aim as practitioners is to bring the patient back to balance. The strength of our medicine is twofold—its energetic paradigm that recognizes patterns of disharmony, as well as the gentle treatment tools we employ.

While a non-specific stress reaction disturbs the flow of energy in the body, a specific stress reaction may involve various *zang fu* organs. These organs are the *yin* organs of the liver, spleen, heart, lung, and kidney. The correct differentiation of signs and symptoms reveals which organs are involved. Stress can lead to symptoms of stagnation, particularly of the blood, because stress, as it consumes *yin*, causes stagnation. Various acupuncture points may be selected for treatment based upon proper discernment of the pattern of disharmony, with the generalized aim of treatment to move the blood, to strengthen the organs, and redistribute and balance the *qi*.

In my experience with general anxiety, post-traumatic stress and episodic anxiety, I have found that there is room for the judicious use of Western medications for the initial phase of shock and stabilization, the therapeutic advice of stress experts, and the unsurpassed effectiveness of acupuncture for rebalancing the patient's energy and promoting recovery.

Certainly as practitioners, we need to balance treating what we see with doing no harm, so there is no set formula for treatment. Treatments should be conservative, for instance using few needles because of the delicacy of the person's presentation. My preferred point selection includes the ones that follow in Table 4.**1**. Due to the nature of the problem being addressed, that is, stress and

Points	Energetics	Locations	Needle Technique
HT-7 (*shen men*)	Heart 7, the earth point and sedation point of the heart channel. It quiets the heart, calms the spirit, and puts the patient into a state of receptivity for treatment	Standard Chinese location—in the depression at the wrist crease between the pisiform and the ulna bones on the radial side of the tendon of the flexor carpi ulnaris muscle. See alternative location, Fig. 3.**3** in Chapter 3	Puncture perpendicularly 0.3 in
SP-6 (*san yin jiao*)	As group *luo* of the three-leg *yin* (liver, spleen, and kidney), SP-6 nourishes the *yin* of the entire body. It regulates the blood	Standard Chinese location—3 *cun* above the tip of the medial malleolus, on the posterior border of the fibula, on the line drawn from the medial malleolus to SP-9 (*yin ling quan*)	Puncture perpendicularly 0.3–0.5 in. Contraindicated in pregnancy
Yin tang	As the reflex point of the pituitary gland, it regulates the blood. By doing so, it controls hormonal secretions and the chemical composition of the blood. It calms the spirit and promotes relaxation. It is the so-called "happy point" for these reasons	Standard Chinese location—in the center of the glabella, between the medial ends of the eyebrows	Puncture subcutaneously and transversely downward (toward the nose) with a threading technique 0.5–0.8 in
GV-20 (*bai hui*)	Awakens the brain, strengthens the brain as a Sea of Marrow. Opens the orifices, clears the mind, stabilizes the will, and purifies the spirit. Expels liver wind, spreads liver *qi*, and restores collapsed *yang*. Regulates the *qi* of the heart. Clears heat, stops spasm	Standard Chinese location—5 *cun* within the anterior hairline on the mid-point that connects the apexes of the two auricles	Puncture subcutaneously and transversely anteriorly (toward the nose) 0.3–0.5 in
KI-1 (*yong quan*)	As the sedation point, tonifies *yin*, clears heat, subdues wind, and empty heat, clears the brain, restores consciousness. Suppresses the liver, regulates blood to the upper part of the body	Standard Chinese location—on the sole of the foot, when the foot is in plantar flexion, the point is located at the upper third and middle two-thirds of the sole, Fig. 4.**1**	Massage deeply or puncture gently with a #1 Seirin needle 0.3–0.5 in
KI-16 (*huang shu*)	Strengthens root *qi*, tonifies the kidney, connects to the heart. Tonifies the spleen because it is close to the navel and the navel corresponds to the earth element; earth is mother of lung and grandmother of kidney so it strengthens them as well	Japanese location—0.5 *cun* all around the center of the umbilicus	Puncture obliquely 0.5–1.0 in towards the navel

Table 4.**1** Point energetics and locations of points to treat anxiety disorders

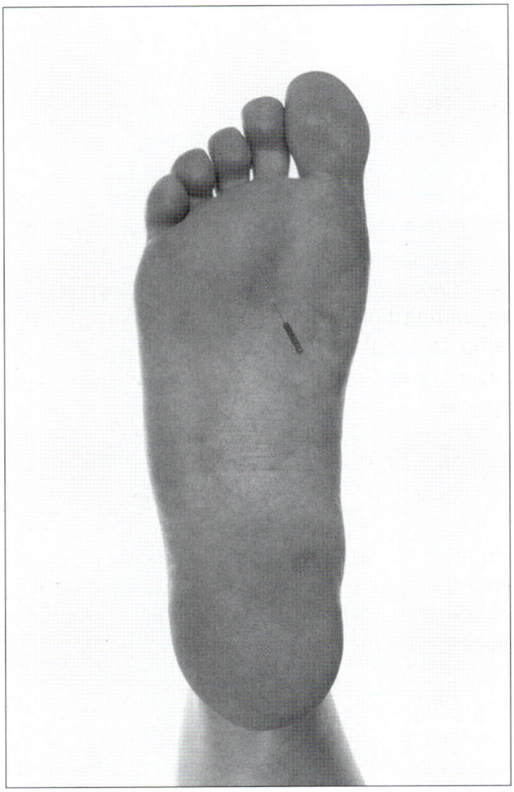

Fig. 4.1 Location of Kidney 1 (*yong quan*). Courtesty of Seirin Europe/3B Scientific, Hamburg, Germany.

anxiety, and for patient comfort, use #1 30 mm Seirin needles. Needles are retained for 10 to 15 minutes.

In summary, Oriental medicine has tremendous clinical relevance for the normal stress of daily life as well as the inordinate stresses of the 21st century that create these serious disorders. It is efficacious physically and psychologically, yet at the same time gentle, and nourishes the deepest level of our existence, the spirit.

Reference

1. Larre P, Rochat de la Vallee E. *Rooted in Spirit.* Barrytown, New York: Station Hill Press; 1995: 4–5

5 The Relationship between Bunions, Sugar, and the Spleen

A bunion, according to Western pathology, is an abnormal prominence on the foot in the inner aspect of the first metatarsal head with bursa formation and fluid accumulation. Etiologies include postural problems such as variation in the position of the first metatarsal because of excessive rolling of the ankles (or pronation of the foot), trauma to the local area, shoes that are too small, osteoarthritis or rheumatic arthritis of the big toe. Other mechanical problems may also affect hallucis longus, the big toe.

The treatment of bunions, as well osteoarthritis of the first metatarsophalangeal joint, with Oriental medical modalities is a curious clinical adaptation to an age-old problem. Bunions can be exceedingly painful for patients who suffer from them, and many do, although perhaps not as a major complaint to the acupuncturist because the patients may not know the benefits of acupuncture for this condition. Typically, patients report discomforting tenderness of the toes. There may be slight swelling of the joint, and shoes may aggravate the patient's condition. As the problem becomes more chronic, pain tends to worsen and joint motion may become limited.

In Japanese acupuncture, bunions or osteoarthritis of the big toe are referred to as "sugar toes." They are so named because the theory behind their appearance is that excess sugar consumption, caused by the failure of the spleen to transform and transport sugar in foods, results in damp. The damp then leads to the formation of phlegm. The phlegm congeals such that an actual bony deformation appears.

Note that the bunion is bordered on either side of the first metatarsal bone by acupuncture points. Distally SP-2 (*da du*) and proximally SP-3 (*tai bai*) are involved. Spleen 2 is the fire point and the tonification point of the spleen, and as such is used to treat spleen vacuity such as the failure of the spleen to transform and transport the sugar, aka the damp. As its earth point and horary point, Spleen 3 balances and strengthens the spleen, stabilizes insulin production and benefits diabetic disharmonies. Sugar can be viewed energetically as both hot and damp, and hence we are not surprised to see the occurrence of corresponding hot (painful, red, and inflamed) and damp (toe enlargement or fluid accumulation) pathology at these points, such as the congealed phlegm.

The typical Western treatment usually begins with physical therapy and local injections. Surgical removal of the bunion may then be recommended. This treatment is not only expensive and painful, but is usually ineffective. The bunion may reoccur because the underlying causes of sugar consumption and metabolism problems have not been addressed. Now the toe may become even more painful because of the trauma of local surgery. Additionally, the creation of a scar, along the spleen channel, may further inhibit the functional role of the spleen as the scar interrupts the *qi* and blood flow of the channel.

Remember that the Oriental view of a scar is that it is a "potential" organ/channel disturbance. What this means is that any scar may lead to the development of pathology on the associated channel, and even more distally to the organ, because its presence may interfere with the flow of *qi* and blood. Whether the scar is actually clinically significant is ultimately determined by palpation of its discrete borders. Objective factors related to appearance, such as discoloration, swelling within or beyond its borders, and oozing, may be an indication that the scar is problematic. The patient may experience criteria such as pain, pulling, itching, numbness, heat, cold, distention, referred sensation, emptiness, or weird feelings. The criteria are usually correlated with some disturbance of *qi* and blood in the area. Palpation is a reliable methodology to determine if the scar is clinically significant, and if so, it should be treated.

Invariably, patients I have seen with bunion problems have had one of the following illnesses relating to sugar history: diabetes, hypoglycemia, and sensitivity to sugar, sugar cravings, sugar allergies, pancreatic cancer, or leaky gut syndrome.

Some have come to see me with these problems as a major complaint, some have not. But in the course of a physical exam, I would notice the bunion on all patients who had these disorders. Seeing this I would then ask them if they craved sugar, if they ate sugar excessively, or if they felt that they had a problem metabolizing sugar, or were hypoglycemic or diabetic, or if these disorders ran in their family. All would affirm some connection with sugar, and they would look incredulously at me, wondering how I knew their secret cravings! At that point I would explain to them what sugar toes were, and provide them with treatment options.

My preferred treatment of this disorder is, locally at least, very simple, effective and fast. There are three major treatment modalities to choose from and they are described below in Table 5.**1**. Figure 5.**1** depicts sugar toe pathology. For those who may not be familiar with this tool, Figure 5.**2** illustrates the tiger thermie warmer (the smaller instrument in the photograph), the lion thermie warmer, and the moxa used in them. There are two forms in the Appendix that describe how to use the tiger thermie warmer and the Chinese liniment *Zheng Gu Shui* respectively. Copies of these may be made and given to patients so they know how to use the tools correctly.

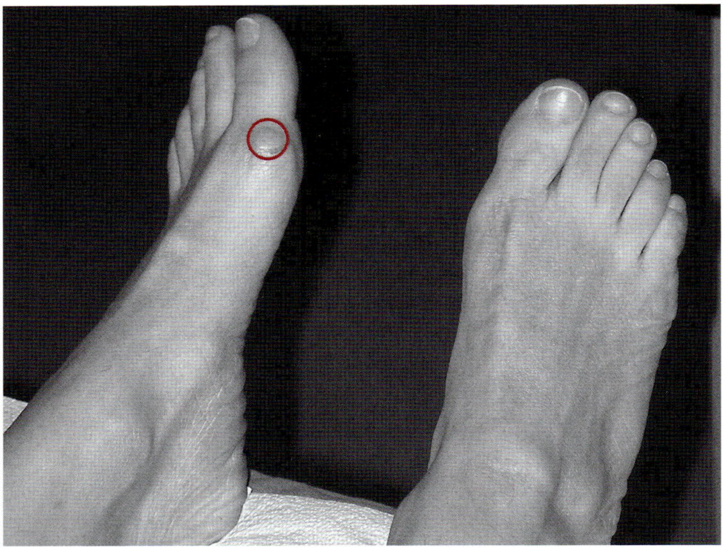

Fig. 5.**1** Sugar toe pathology (see circle).

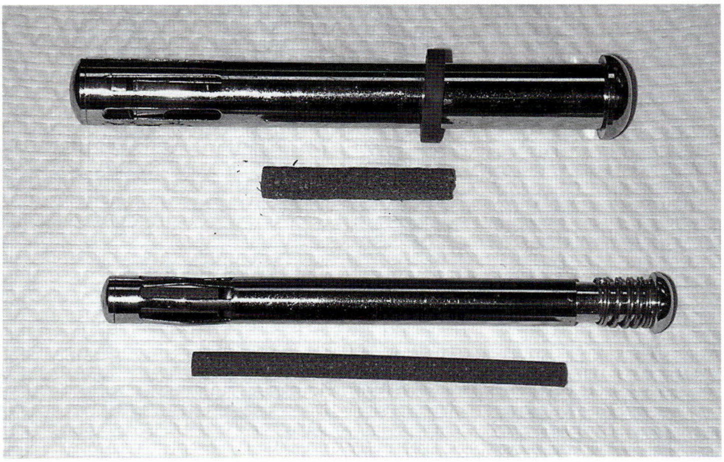

Fig. 5.**2** The lion thermie warmer (top), the tiger thermie warmer and moxa.

Modality	Rationale	Method
1. *Zheng Gu Shui* liniment This is my modality of choice. I sell it to the patient and have them use it daily. Provide written instructions for use (see Appendix for form to photocopy)	*Zheng Gu Shui* (Royal Bone Water) is the hottest of the Chinese liniments. By virtue of this it penetrates through the skin, muscle, and channels, all the way to the bone level, which is where and what the bunion is. The liniment breaks up the calcium deposits and arthritic bone deformities of the bunions. It disperses blood, fluid, and *qi* stagnation and thereby stops pain	Wet a cotton ball generously with *Zheng Gu Shui*. Apply liberally to the entire area of the bunion. Let it dry and repeat again. In particular, put on before bed, but it may be used anytime. Do not bandage or cover tightly; it will cause serious burns. Do not heat the liniment up. Do not apply with massage. Avoid all mucous membranes. *Zheng Gu Shui* is flammable and can stain clothing. Do not apply if the area is hot and swollen
2. Tiger thermie warmer The combined use of the tiger thermie warmer and *Zheng Gu Shui* is especially valuable. Apply the liniment according to the directions listed above. Let it dry. Then use the tiger thermie warmer as directed. Use daily or several times per week. Sell the patient the tiger thermie warmer and provide written instructions for the patient (see Appendix for form to photocopy)	A Japanese moxa instrument used to deliver the therapeutic benefits of moxa (which penetrates deeply to the channel level), and by way of its usage breaks up channel obstructions	Pull the tiger thermie warmer apart. Insert a stick of moxa in the clip of the handle. Place the cap back on and make sure the tip of the moxa is in the vented area of the cap. If it is not, readjust it, otherwise the moxa will not burn effectively Take the cap back off and light the moxa stick. Gently blowing on it will help it get going and stay lit. As the moxa burns down, move the body of the tiger thermie warmer such that the moxa is in the optimal burning position, i.e., in the vented part of the cap. When applying the moxa put the warm tip to the skin; be careful not to get it too hot. Check it often and adjust as needed. You can adjust the burning tip for more warmth and/or to cool off the tip Use light stroking motions on SP-2 and SP-3. A gradual warming of the point is best. Start slowly, move gently, and give the moxa time to warm the area. Going too slow can result in the skin getting hot too quickly and cause a burn. In case of a bunion, heat each point, Spleen 2 and 3, for 1 minute on each point by touching the point with the tiger thermie warmer, removing it and retouching it
3. Needles	To invigorate stagnation locally and activate the function of the spleen to transform and transport	Needle SP-2 and SP-3 perpendicularly 0.1 – 0.2 in and 0.5 – 0.1 in respectively with an even technique. Needling is tender due to the points' locations on the side of the foot. Patients may prefer *Zheng Gu Shui* due to the ease of application on a daily basis. Needles require an office visit, cost more, and are more invasive, but of course they work too

Table 5.**1** The clinical treatment of sugar toes

Note that although the local area characterized by the bunion is treated, the acupuncture points work on the regulation of the spleen due to their energetics. Other acupuncture points, based upon signs and symptoms, and differentiated by syndrome, can be chosen to augment the treatment that you are providing for the patient.

If the bunion is due to the presence of phlegm (versus a postural or mechanical problem), and the patient treats him/herself frequently with the tiger thermie warmer and *Zheng Gu Shui* liniment, immediate improvement in pain should be noted in one week. Even decreased sensitivity to sugar can ensue and the patient may be able to eat such products with no further problems because the spleen has been strengthened. Shrinking of the bunion typically occurs and continues to do so, especially with the adjunct application of the Chinese liniment, *Zheng Gu Shui*.

6 An Oriental Medical Physician's Framework for the Understanding and Treatment of Cancer

Within any paradigm, for any practitioner, an understanding of cancer and its treatment is a formidable prospect. Voluminous information has, must and certainly will continue to be written about it. In this chapter, I aim to provide the practitioner of Oriental medicine with a basic outline and a general thinking approach to the pathophysiology and treatment of cancer for clinical use.

Millions of people throughout the world have been stricken with cancer's devastating and life-threatening varieties. For the most part, the standard Western treatment entails the equally devastating treatments of chemotherapy or radiation. As with many diseases, the strength of allopathic (conventional) medicine is its specificity of knowledge at the molecular level, and the strength of Oriental medicine its ability to frame physiological processes and treatment plans in general terms. This complementary contrast becomes apparent when addressing the topic of cancer.

The powerful tools of Oriental medicine can be successfully applied to cancer patients, not so much to treat the cancer per se, but to treat the ravaging side-effects of its standard therapy. In doing so, not only are these side-effects diminished, but the vital energy of the whole person is also enhanced, resulting in general improvement in their quality of life.

This chapter is divided into two parts—the etiology and pathophysiology of cancer from Western and Oriental perspectives and then its treatment from those perspectives. Insight into its pathogenesis is important in providing valuable clues for treatment, be it with surgery, chemicals, acupuncture, or herbs and these options are all explored.

■ Cancer in Western and Oriental Medicine: Etiology and Pathophysiology

Unrestrained Tissue Growth

Normal healthy cells live in a complex, interdependent environment, regulating one another's proliferation. Continual reproduction of cells is a natural part of life, however, there must be specific mechanisms to prevent any particular type of cell from reproducing to the maximum extent its environment will permit. In the adult body, cells are regulated in such a way as to maintain the size, shape, and functions of the tissues and structures of the body. Normally, the cells of the body multiply and divide in a gradual and orderly fashion. They respect each other's boundaries and only grow when other cells wear out and die. Cancer cells however, will continue to grow right over each other and over healthy cells and can suffocate normal cells with their aggressive growth and overcrowding.

The regulating mechanism of the cell is its DNA. DNA is coding material, which, among other things, guides the cell in the manufacture of new components. There are many mechanisms that cause mutation of DNA and the breakdown in the normal control of cellular reproduction that it directs. The full range of these causative factors is not known, but certainly there are chemical agents that appear responsible for certain cases, such as tumors. Emotional factors may play a part, perhaps by modulating hormone levels. Toxins and viruses may also be implicated. In some cases, sunlight damages the DNA.

The following factors likewise appear to be possible causes of cancer: chronic electromagnetic field exposure; genetic mutation; chronic stress; sick building syndrome; ionizing/nuclear radiation; pesticide/herbicide residues; industrial toxins; polluted water, chlorinated water, fluorinated water; tobacco and smoking; immune-suppressing drugs; irradiated foods, food additives, nutritional deficiencies; mercury toxicity, dental factors; nerve interference; depressed thyroid function; intestinal toxicity and digestive impairment, parasites; blocked detoxification pathways; free radicals; cellular oxygen deficiency/cellular terrain, oncogene, genetic predisposition and miasm.

The Harvard School of Public Health claims that other co-morbid factors that could reduce 2.5 million of the 7 million deaths per year in the United States alone due to cancer include smoking, alcohol, lack of exercise, diet, unsafe sex, contaminated needles, and obesity.

Stages of Growth

Not only do cancer cells ignore the usual controls and proliferate according to their own agenda, they also have the ability to migrate from the original site and invade nearby tissue. The resulting mass of new tissue forms a tumor, which is called a neoplasm. The pathology of cancer proceeds according to the following stages:

1. Tumor development begins when a cell within a normal population sustains a genetic mutation that increases its propensity to proliferate when it would normally rest. DNA repair genes that make proteins to correct errors may fail to do their job. Also, the presence or absence of repressor genes may not regulate cell multiplication.
2. The altered cell and its descendants continue to look normal, but they reproduce too much—a condition termed hyperplasia. After years, one in a million of these cells undergoes another mutation that further loosens control on cell growth.
3. In addition to proliferating excessively, the offspring of the altered cell appear abnormal in shape and in orientation; the tissue is now said to exhibit dysplasia. Once again, after a time, a rare mutation occurs that alters cell behavior.
4. The affected cells become still more abnormal in growth and appearance. If the tumor has not yet broken through any boundaries between tissues, it is called in situ cancer. This tumor may remain contained indefinitely, however, some cells may eventually acquire mutations.
5. If the genetic changes allow the tumor to begin invading underlying tissue and to shed cells into the blood or lymph, the mass is considered to have become malignant. The renegade cells are likely to establish new tumors (metastases) throughout the body via the blood system or the lymphatic system. The metastases may become lethal by disrupting a vital organ. Some cancers are more likely to metastasize than others. Melanoma often spreads to the lungs. Colon or rectal cancer frequently spreads to the liver and prostate cancer to the bones.
6. Locally, in a process called angiogenesis, new blood vessels may be formed when the malignant cells secrete chemicals that create a new blood supply for the tumor. With access to a steady source of nutrients, the tumor can grow indefinitely.

Types of Cancer

Many different types of cancer have three features common:

1. The cancerous tissues have the ability for continuous, indefinite proliferation.
2. The tumor may invade surrounding normal tissue.
3. The cancer has the tendency to spread throughout the body if it disengages from the primary tumor, travels through the circulatory system, and establishes colonies at distant sites.

Some tumors are benign; some are malignant. Benign tumors have an expansible growth pattern, enlarging locally within their host structures. They are usually contained within a capsule and do not spread to distant sites. Their cells are fairly well differentiated and cell turnover is slower. Malignant tumors on the other hand have an invasive growth pattern—over-running host stroma and other tissue structures. They can invade body cavities and blood and lymph channels, spreading to secondary sites (metastasis). Their cell replication is rapid and frequently abnormal. Poor differentiations and maturation of cells are typical, including a tendency to regress to a pre-differentiated or ancestor-type cell (anaplasia).[1]

- From a Western perspective there are some common signs and symptoms that suggest cancer[2], although due to the lack of a substantive mass in the early stages, pain may not be a symptom:
  - There may be a tendency to hemorrhage,

which indicates a breakthrough of the malignancy.
- Clotting abnormalities, reduced or increased, may occur.
- The patient may be subject to infection or have an immunosuppressed disorder.
- It may be characterized by puzzling tissue damage or poor resolution of injury or illness.
- Fever, without other signs or symptoms, may be present.
- The patient may experience cachexia (marked weight loss and wasting tissue), accompanied by loss of appetite and malabsorption of nutrients, as well as nausea, vomiting, and diarrhea.
- Abnormal hormonal secretion can occur.
- Red skin lesions or a purple rash can develop.
- Nervous system complications are common, as well as disorders of vital organs such as the brain, liver, heart, kidney, and lungs.

Chinese medicine recognizes a number of imbalances that contribute to the formation of cancer. It is primarily viewed as due to two leading pathological factors—stagnant blood and phlegm. Sometimes stagnant blood and phlegm may co-exist. They are also capable of engendering each other. Almost any stimulus may lead to the development of stagnant blood and phlegm. The most common include those listed below[3]:

- Disharmony of *qi* and blood, which leads to stagnation.
- Development of and stagnation of phlegm.
- Invasion by evil toxins. (In allopathic medicine this would include carcinogenic factors and viruses.)
- Kidney and spleen deficiencies—pre- and postnatal *qi* deficiencies. (These could be viewed as Western genetic factors.)
- The seven emotions or internal causes of disease (anger, joy, fear, fright, grief, anxiety, and thought [worry]).
- The external causes of disease (evil *qi*)—wind, cold, damp, dryness, heat, summer heat. (These can also be subsumed under viruses and carcinogenic factors.)
- The neutral causes of disease such as dietary irregularities of excessive drinking and ingestion of cold, hot, and greasy food, alcohol, and foods that lead to phlegm formation.

Since blood stagnation and phlegm are seen as two of the major contributing factors, the following are the corresponding treatment principles most commonly utilized when treating cancer by traditional Chinese medicine[4]:

- regulate the *qi* and harmonize blood to resolve the stasis to maintain unobstructed flow of the channels and collaterals;
- transform phlegm and eliminate damp;
- soften the hard and dissolve nodules;
- dissolve toxins and stop pain;
- tonify *qi* and cultivate blood;
- invigorate the spleen and pacify the stomach;
- replenish and tonify the liver and kidneys.

The opinions of leading physicians in literature are useful to review to provide insight for the practitioner on how to apply these principles. Physician Ru Jin Zhao's approach to the treatment of cancer lies in "adjusting the macroenvironment to adjust the microenvironment (the body)." He maintains that phlegm formation is a major mechanism in the development of cancer. Therefore, his approach is to treat the lungs to alleviate the development of substantial phlegm formation and to promote stomach *yin*, the lack of which contributes to phlegm formation.[5]

Zhang Dai-Zhao, author of *The Treatment of Cancer by Integrated Chinese-Western Medicine*[6] claims, "Treat the branch in acute cases and treat the root in chronic cases." The root implies supporting the righteous *qi* and eliminating evil *qi* at the same time. For him, this means giving large quantities of herbs to tonify and benefit the *qi* and blood in order to promote fortification of the patient, and the administration of both Western and Chinese anti-cancerous substances to prevent recurrence and metastasis. He says, "The severity of the condition and the stage of the disease must be thoroughly understood when administering Chinese herbal ingredients. There is a saying in TCM, 'Cracking toxins with poisons.' The treatment of cancer in general proceeds from the principle of cracking toxins with poisons. However, if special attention is not paid to the overall condition of the patient, random cracking always results in early deterioration and death."[7]

The warning here is that focus should be on addressing the whole person by supporting their *zheng qi* (true or righteous *qi*), even while "attacking" the cancer. A correlation is easily drawn here between the Chinese idea of "Cracking toxins with poisons" and the Western idea of chemotherapy and radiation.

Others purport that cancer, like all other diseases, is regarded as the underlying imbalance. The tumor is the uppermost branch, not the root of the illness.[8] It is generally recognized that cancer is a local manifestation of a general ailment. Once a tumor mass exists, there will be manifestations of *yin–yang* disharmony.[9]

In *The Practice of Chinese Medicine*[10], Giovanni Maciocia states, "Abdominal masses cannot be separated from that of Western diagnosis. In the case of abdominal masses perhaps more than any other, a Western diagnosis is essential. We should never treat them blindly without first establishing what they really are. This is because masses in the abdomen can be due to a number of causes, including enlarged organs, cysts, myomas, spastic colon, fecal masses, or tumors."

In *Treating Cancer with Chinese Herbs*, herbalist Hong-Yen Hsu posits, "In Chinese medicine, diagnosis of tumors is made through the four methods: observing, listening, questioning, and palpating. Through these methods, the *Yin* or *Yang*, surface or inside, chill or fever, weak or firm conformations, existence, or non-existence of pus, and hence the malignancy or benignity of the cancer are noted. Then after summarizing the data, a correct judgement can be made."[11]

From the Chinese medical view that the causative factor comes under the heading of "toxin," a concept that inherently implies a vigorous pathogen, which usually localizes its impact. What causes the growth to persist over a prolonged time is the alteration of normal blood circulation. The tissues are unable to return to normal because the blood can no longer help to organize the normal pattern of growth and breakdown. The treatment for the excessive growth is normalization of blood circulation and elimination of the toxin. It is often thought that the blood vitalizing is the critical factor because once the circulation is normalized there is a chance for the body to eliminate the toxin on its own.

Finally, the renowned C.S. Cheung's treatment strategy maintains that in its early stages the cancer is an excess, and so the excess or branch should be addressed. In the mid to latter stages, the patient presents with a combined repletion/vacuity pattern with emphasis on vacuity and so should treatment. In the later stages, characterized by further vacuity, the treatment plan should be to support the normal *qi* and reduce pain. He considers it critical to treat according to differentiation of the pattern, not the Western 'type' of cancer. He says it is important to perform tongue diagnosis to assist in the proper differentiation in order to select acupuncture and herbs for treatment.[12]

As suggested by all of these sources, it is important to be aware of the root and branch of the disease, as well as the severity of the condition, the stage of disease and location of the cancer as determined by Western diagnostic tools so as to formulate a treatment plan.

■ Integrated Cancer Treatment Modalities—Western and Chinese

An integrated approach to the treatment of cancer, using both Western and Chinese medicines, is a solid, rational, and recommended approach. The Western treatment truly uses an "attack" principle of treating cancer (the Chinese idea of cracking toxins with poisons), which, in turn, produces many debilitating side-effects. It is essentially in the treatment of these side-effects that Chinese medicine excels. In addition to treating the symptoms of such side-effects, Chinese herbal therapy also treats the root by supporting the *zheng qi*, improving immunity, and decreasing the percentage of recurrence.

Chinese Herbs in the Management of Cancer

Herbal formulas constitute the primary form of treating cancer with TCM. In China, the majority of cancer patients are treated by Western therapies, although the selection of drugs used in chemotherapy is frequently different due to approval of new compounds in China not yet used in the West. There are two basic situations, described below, where herbal therapies enter into cancer treatment.

As we have seen, the term cancer applies to a wide range of diseases, which have, as a common factor, the loss of normal cellular growth control mechanisms. Most cancers manifest symptoms of "accumulation," described in traditional Chinese medicine terms as entanglement of *qi*, stasis of blood, and accumulation of phlegm. While each cancer type deserves independent study and treatment, and though each patient will have different constitutional factors that influence the specific treatment, there exist general principles of herb therapy that can be applied to most cancer patients.

Herbs that are more specific to the tumor type being treated, and in several cases *qi* tonics, are added to enhance immunity and benefit the weakened patient. The features of the herbal approach are described below:

- Herbs can nourish the kidney and liver, and regulate the circulation of *qi* and blood.
- Herbs can influence the hormonal system.
- Chinese herbal therapy is used to make the individual healthier.
- Chinese herbal therapy is used to keep estrogen at the level the body needs, which is at a moderate level. The Western medical approach is to ensure no further tumor growth by keeping estrogen low. One cannot ensure that herbs will not influence estrogen. Chinese herbs may very well be of benefit to the individual who has had an estrogen-dependent tumor. However, they should not be used in cases where estrogenic materials are strictly prohibited by the oncologist. It is therefore recommended that patients wishing to follow their oncologist's recommendation about estrogen do not use any Chinese herbs.

  Licorice (*Radix Glycyrrhizae*) is purported to have estrogenic activity. The main activity of licorice, in terms of hormones, is a corticosteroid-like anti-inflammatory action. Small doses of licorice (or its main active component glycyrrhizin and glycyrrhetinic acid) have been shown in laboratory animals to reduce the action of estrogen on growth of the uterus (thus antagonizing estrogen effects), but high doses (much higher than in Chinese herbal formulas) were found to potentiate the action of estrogen. These components have been shown in other studies to lower estrogenic activity when it is high and potentiate it when it is low. Thus, if anything, it is possible that licorice has a protective effect. Further, active components from licorice, such as glycyrrhetinic acid, have been shown to have anti-tumor activity.
- Herbs can assist the chemotherapeutic agent in destroying the tumor. Prescriptions with a large number of ingredients in the form of an herbal decoction are provided in Chinese hospitals to address both the tumor site and the general problem of "resolving" the swelling. The use of a tumor-reducing herbal compounds becomes more important if the oncologist believes that chemotherapy alone has a limited chance of eliminating the tumor (based on statistics from previous attempts).
- Anti-tumor formulas, usually adjusted to the type of cancer being treated, are also administered in the hope of causing a more rapid and complete elimination of the tumor. Studies conducted in China indicate about a 50 % increase in average survival time in cases of lung or liver tumors when herbal therapies are used. Similar prescriptions may be used in persons who do not undertake any of the Western therapies because they are deemed ineffective or undesirable for some reason. A few hospitals in China specialize in the treatment of cancer using mostly herbal therapies.
- Herbs are used to counteract the side-effects of anti-cancer therapies. They are used to decrease nausea and other gastrointestinal distress or to reduce leukopenia and other blood disorders that arise. Herbs are also used to offset the immune-suppressing action of chemotherapy.

Fu Zheng Pei Ben (FZPB) is an herbal treatment currently used in China in the integrated treatment of cancer.[13] The main principles of *Fu Zheng Pei Ben* are to:

- prevent the formation and development of cancer;
- increase immunity;
- enhance the regulating functions of the endocrine and humoral systems;
- protect the bone marrow and promote its hematopoietic function;
- strengthen digestion and absorption and improve metabolism;

- rectify deviation of *yin–yang* relations;
- increase the effects of all therapeutic measures of Western medicine;
- in addition to herbal treatments, utilizes both nutritional therapy and *qi gong*.

The FZPB materia medica is based on the principles of *yin* and *yang*, *qi* and blood. The herbal categories utilized include *yin*-replenishing herbs, *yang*-reinforcing herbs, *qi*-replenishing herbs, blood tonics or blood-nourishing herbs, pathogenic heat-removing herbs, polysaccharides; blood-replenishing and invigorating herbs; immunological function-enhancing herbs, and herbs for the spleen and stomach that regulate digestion and enhance assimilation of nutrients.

Among the *fu zheng* herbs commonly found in the West are *Astragalus*-based formulas, which contain immune-enhancing polysaccharides, medicinal mushroom products and ginseng-based formulas, which contain saponins that have immune-enhancing effects.[14]

In treating certain cancers with Chinese herbal remedies, in conjunction with chemotherapy and/or radiation, it may be important to include herbs that help raise the count of erythrocytes, leukocytes, and thrombocytes, such as *Radix Pilosulae Codonopsis, Radix Rehmanniae Glutinosae, Radix Angelica Sinensis, Radix Ginseng* and *Radix Salviae Miltiorrhizae*, among others. The components used in the formulas should contain at least one of these herbs. Check with the patient's doctor about this strategy as it can be contraindicated for some cancers.

Surgery

Western Treatment Principle

Surgical removal of tumor.

TCM Treatment Principle—*Fu Zheng Pei Ben* Principle[15]

Prior to the surgery, rectify the deviation of *yin/yang*, that is, strengthen the body for surgery. After surgery, the function of the spleen and stomach should be strengthened, the *yin* nourished, and body fluids promoted for post-operative symptoms of dry mouth, constipation, coughing, fever, and infection.

Chemotherapy

Western Treatment Principle

Chemotherapy is used to treat the systemic nature of metastatic neoplasms. Chemotherapy should only be used:

- To effect a cure—used alone or with other modalities such as surgery and radiation.
- For palliation—to afford significant relief of symptoms and, in certain cases prolong survival. The side-effects of chemotherapy are numerous and, at times, life-threatening, e.g., nausea, vomiting, weight loss, anorexia, diarrhea, abdominal pain, renal tubular damage, decreased kidney size, fibrosis, fatigue, somnolence, confusion, agitation, hallucination, headache, irritability, depression, hypersensitivity, fever, chills, sterility, menopausal symptoms, amenorrhea, alopecia, dermatitis, oral ulcerations, photosensitivity, hyperpigmentation, hemorrhagic and non-hemorrhagic cystitis, pneumonia, elevated transaminases, and hepatitis.

TCM Treatment Principle[16]

Tonify and cultivate *qi*, invigorate the spleen and harmonize the stomach, nourish and tonify the liver and kidneys, and clear heat and dissolve toxins. FZPB therapy prevents, alleviates, and diminishes the side-effects of chemotherapy, and strengthens its actions with herbs containing polysaccharides. When there are only mild side-effects or no side-effects, TCM can be applied. If the side-effects are serious, integrated methods should be used, including blood transfusion for bone marrow inhibition and antibiotics or hormones for infection.

Radiation Therapy

Western Treatment Principle

The goal of radiation therapy is to sterilize a targeted tumor completely while preserving the integrity of surrounding normal structures. Nearly 60 % of all cancer patients undergo radiation therapy either by a beam that is directed toward the tumor area or placement of radioactive sources directly into the malignancy. Side-effects include skin toxicity; oral cavity and mandibular toxicity (decreased salivation); hematologic toxicity (injury to bone marrow, affecting blood production); and gastrointestinal toxicity (nausea, vomiting, diarrhea that commonly occur 2 to 6 hours after abdominal or pelvic irradiation).

TCM Treatment Principle[17]

The side-effects of radiation mostly cause injury to the *yin* fluids by hot toxins, disharmony of the stomach/spleen, and vacuity and injury of the liver and kidneys. Therefore, the following treatment strategies should be considered: clear heat and remove toxins, generate fluids and moisten dryness, cool and tonify *qi* and blood, invigorate spleen and harmonize stomach, and nourish and tonify the liver and kidneys.

According to TCM[18], ionized radiation is an aggressive material with a hot nature, which may become evil fire, consuming body fluid and essence, leading to *yin* vacuity and decreased body resistance. The following FZ treatment principles should also be considered: move blood in order to enhance radiotherapeutic effect by increasing blood circulation, therefore delivery of radiation to the tumor site; nourish the *yin* of the kidney and liver; tonify *qi* and nourish *yin*.

Immunotherapy

Western Treatment Principle

The primary goal of immunotherapy is to recruit the body's natural defense mechanism, the immune system, to combat the malignancy. The process is to administer substances designed to provoke an anti-tumor response by the body's own cells.

TCM Treatment Principle

Nourish the spleen and stomach, nourish the kidneys, harmonize the *qi* and blood, and resolve stasis.

Bone Marrow Transplantation

Western Treatment Principle

Bone marrow transplantation has been proven to be curative in cancers that were previously uniformly fatal. It affords the opportunity to exploit doses of chemotherapy and radiation that normally produce excessive hematological toxicity. Specific complications of bone marrow transplantation include the following: infection; subacute, nonbacterial interstitial pneumonia; hemorrhagic cystitis; veno-occlusive disease of the liver, pulmonary complications (obstructive lung disease); endocrine complications (infertility, hypothyroidism); secondary malignancies.

TCM Treatment Principle

Nourish the spleen and stomach, nourish the kidneys, tonify *qi* and nourish blood, stop bleeding, prevent stasis.

Acupuncture Strategies

An understanding of how cancer spreads has implications for treatment. The ways are summarized below again so that we can see their relationship to acupuncture strategies. Cancer spreads:

- through progressive direct local invasion of nearby structures;
- through body cavities;
- via the blood stream (hematogenous metastasis). Most lethal cancers are this type; and
- via the lymphatic system (lymphogenous metastasis).

The highest risk of metastasis probably occurs from direct contact or other strong stimuli applied on or near a tumor, especially if it is close to the skin. However, the odds of survival of the shedded cells are less than 1%. Even so, practitioners should be aware of these routes of transmission and select treatment modalities accordingly. This would mean not massaging or palpating a tumor. Intense movement modalities and heat application should be limited or avoided. Metastatic sites should be approached with caution. While fears about increasing blood and lymph circulation are probably unfounded, the benefits and risks must be weighed, and informed consent obtained for this as well as any type of treatment.[19]

With its 5000-year history, Chinese medicine has become adept at recognizing the signs and symptoms of the healthy human organism. Likewise, it has developed and refined treatment modalities that redirect, cultivate and maintain proper physiological functioning. The essential Chinese treatment plan for patients who are diagnosed with cancer is to support normal cellular, tissue, and organ physiology in the wake of the ravaging and yet life-saving techniques that characterize the most common allopathic approaches to cancer—surgery, drug therapies, and radiation. Utilizing these standard treatments, augmentation with Chinese medical treatment not only relieves many of the side-effects caused by these therapies, but has also been shown clinically to strengthen the patient from the cellular through the spiritual level.

The Chinese treatment modalities most effective in the treatment of the whole person, and likewise the cancer, include as we have seen, internal and external herbal therapy. Additionally, auricular acupuncture, body acupuncture, moxibustion (a combined heat/herbal therapy) and guided imagery are recommended. Patients respond well to these treatments, many of which are simple to learn, easy to administer, and are both cost and clinically effective because they are based on the Chinese world view that recognizes the patterns of the proper flow of energy (or proper physiology and functioning).

Documented increase in white blood cell production; heightened energy; re-growth of hair; increased libido; decrease in nausea and vomiting; improvement in appetite, decreased abdominal distention, loose stools or constipation; alleviation of depression, anxiety, fear, irritability or other emotional aberrations; quicker wound-healing capacity and response to infection; decrease in skin irritation, dry skin, muscular weakness; regulation of weight loss, thirst, and pain; improvement in respiration—in short, an overall improvement in the quality of life, both in terms of physical and emotional problems and affect—these are the primary signs and symptoms with which Chinese medicine has results. A broad range of systemic clinical manifestations is addressed, but ultimately, through this style of medicine, immunity is enhanced.

Chinese medicine is time-tested, person-oriented and clinically applicable to the devastating illnesses of our time such as cancer. Although ancient, it parallels innovative Western techniques that are being developed to address this difficult disease, with its emphasis on the intimate relationship between the person and the planet, cultural stresses, nutrition and genetic inheritance.

The "secret" to its success lies in its artistry, that is, its ability to view each person as a unique constellation of energy or symptoms, not as a disease. The key to this ability to do so is because, while it certainly recognizes and can categorize and differentiate clinical manifestations into a disease pattern, it never sees the body, mind, and spirit as separate. Fundamentally, the preponderance of symptoms are viewed as rooted in spirit, and as the primary Chinese medical text the *Huang Di Nei Jing* (*The Yellow Emperor's Classic of Medicine*) reminds us "In order to cure disease, one must first establish contact with a patient's spirit."

Such complementary therapies should be sought out for the benefit of each individual patient and is consonant with the general goals of the Cancer Advisory Panel on Complementary and Alternative Medicine (CAPCAM), the National Cancer Institute (NCI) and undoubtedly any physician's deepest desires.

Over the last 25 years, I have treated cancer patients both in my private practice, as well as during a 1-year externship at a Western facility that I headed up for the students at my college. The following treatments were used successfully with those patients, not to cure them, but to assist in improving the quality of their lives while undergoing Western therapeutics. Measurement of the effectiveness of cancer treatment is usually considered successful if there is first an improved sense of well-being. Most patients reported this feeling as early as their first treatment and this was certainly the strength of the medicine we had to offer them. Within limits, increased weight gain and increased white blood cell production is usually desirable. The results of Western tests are, of course, necessary to determine cure.

Auricular Medicine

The first treatment, which I devised to treat patients and have the students use in this fast-paced Western oncology clinic, involved auriculotherapy. Due to the unique nature of this clinical setting we began with a quick, easy-to-do treatment of utilizing auricular acupuncture on these patients. This modality was selected for its non-invasiveness and its quick-acting and long-term effectiveness.

A core prescription was designed with the combined purposes of addressing both the side-effects of allopathic treatment, the nature of the illness, and the person as a whole. It was employed in numerous ways—in its essence as described here, as the skeletal outline of the treatment where points

Point	Energetics
1. *Shen men*	Perhaps the most important point in this prescription. *Shen men* is used to quiet the heart, calm the spirit, and ground the patient. It puts the patient into a state of receptivity for treatment by establishing contact with the patient's spirit. According to the ancient *Su Wen* text, "when the heart is serene, all pain is negligible." *Shen men* regulates the blood as it pertains to the heart. It reduces insomnia, anxiety, palpitations, neurasthenia, and restlessness—common symptoms related to radiation and chemotherapy treatment. It neutralizes toxins, and cures inflammations, side-effects of Western therapy
2. Sympathetic (any of its three locations)	It decreases pain by increasing vasodilation, improves circulation, supports the sympathetic nervous system, and balances the autonomic nervous system, thereby improving overall functioning. It addresses the pain that is usually a symptom of cancer treatment therapies
3. Lung (upper or lower)	As the master of the *qi*, it increases energy, improves respiration, and sends its energy to the kidney to further assist in respiration. It moves the liver (metal controls wood), thus assisting in pain relief, relieves depression, strengthens *wei qi* (defense *qi*) functioning and improves oxygenation. It aids in skin problems such as decreased wound-healing capacity, and decreases dry and irritated skin caused by Western cancer therapies
4. Liver	Promotes the free-flowingness of *qi*, maintains the internal patency of *qi*, and regulates the relationship between the internal and external environment. It moves *qi* and blood that may be stagnant and balances the emotions. There is usually a large emotional component to cancer and its treatment. It builds *yin* and blood that are consumed with radiation
5. Kidney	It tonifies the root *qi*, the basis of our immunity. It assists in hair regrowth and increases libido—problems cancer patients can experience
6–7. Spleen and stomach	To reinforce the *qi* of the central burner (for nausea, vomiting; assists in digestion, improves appetite). They reduce damp/phlegm, thereby reducing thirst, and abdominal distention. They control the blood and the blood vessels. As earth points, they ground the patient, strengthen muscles and build blood
8. Brain (also known as sub-cortex)	For fatigue, anxiety, swelling, shock, etc. It regulates cerebral excitation and pain perception. Regulates all body systems and all neurological functioning. Reduces inflammation. Because it benefits the mind it can be used for insomnia and neuropsychiatric disorders accompanying the illness

Note: If needed, add or delete points based upon signs and symptoms.

Table 6.**1** Ear acupuncture treatment for oncology patients

could be added or deleted, or in combination with other treatments. These points and their energetic functions are described below and in Table 6.**1**. Their locations are also illustrated in Figure 6.**1**.

Needles and Magrain pellets were most commonly employed. For patients whose constitution was relatively stronger or for those who could not have body acupuncture (for instance, they could not lie down comfortably or a room was not available) 36 gauge ear needles in contrast to the normal 28 g used for the ear, chosen for patient comfort, were inserted in one ear to the standard depths of insertion (approximately 0.01 *cun*). A strong stimulus obtained by twirling was performed and the needles were retained 15 to 30 minutes. The opposite ear was then reinforced with pellets so that the patient could continue to receive the benefit of treatment.

For needle-sensitive or weakened patients, gold Magrain pellets, chosen for their tonifying effects and ease of application were affixed to the ear for 3 to 5 days. Patients were instructed to gently

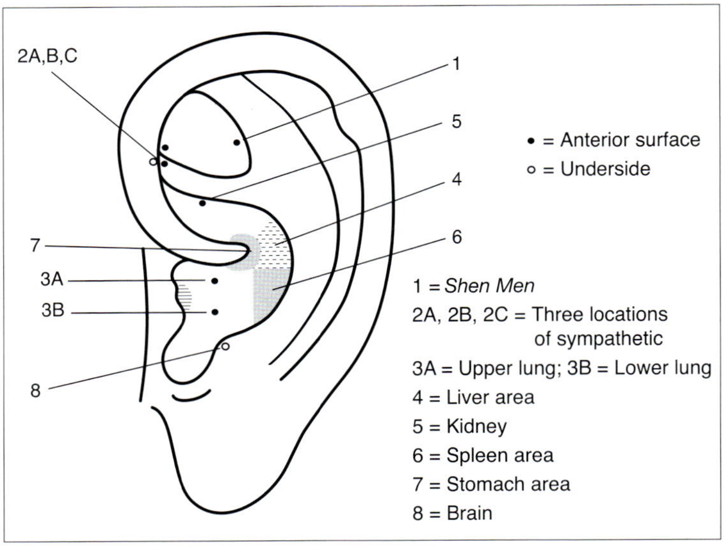

Fig. 6.**1** Location of auricular points for oncology patients.

massage the pellets for about 3 to 5 seconds several times a day and return to the clinic or remove them if they could not come in for a treatment since the possibility of ear infection is possible in patients who already are immunocompromised. Regardless of the type of cancer, patients' response to this method of treatment was favorable. Most reported an abatement of symptoms such as nausea and fatigue and an improvement in appetite, sleep, stools, stamina, and emotional attitude. On those on whom it worked best, patients would report they could tell the difference between having the pellets in or out of their ear. They always felt better with them in.

This simple yet effective treatment plan can be used to assist such patients in not only managing the devastating symptoms of chemotherapy or radiation so the quality of daily living is improved, but simultaneously augment the vital *qi* of the body, which is the basis of all health.

Eight Needle Technique

Another treatment strategy I adopted is a formula I learned on my first externship to China in 1988 called eight needle technique. The Chinese specify that this strategy is for low back pain due to kidney *qi* and *yang* vacuity, and it certainly is. However, an analysis of its points illustrate that it can be used to tonify the kidney, the root *qi* of the body, and the source of both pre-natal and post-natal *qi*—what, in a nutshell, could be called our immunity. Consequently, by treating kidney *qi* and *yang* vacuity there is a broad range of clinical applicability to this formula. I use it this way with excellent result. Table 6.**2** outlines the points used in that strategy, their locations and angles and depths of insertion and energetics. The energetics of the points are discussed below.

As the back *shu* point of kidney, BL-23 (*shen shu*) tonifies and regulates the *qi* of the kidney. It is good for strengthening the kidney's reception of *qi* in the case of respiratory ailments. It is good for chronic eye disorders such as blurred vision, weak legs, and irregular menses. It resolves dampness in the lower burner and strengthens the lower back.

Bladder 23 is better for tonifying the *yang* aspect of kidney *qi*, but it can also be used for kidney *yin* vacuity. Consequently, it can be used for *yang* pathologies such as lack of sexual desire, lack of will power, lack of initiative, depression, dizziness, poor memory, fatigue, constant desire to sleep, cold knees, renal colic, and nephritis. *Yin* vacuity symptoms it can treat include tidal fever and seizures.

Bladder 23 nourishes kidney essence making the point useful in impotence, nocturnal emissions, infertility and spermatorrhea. It benefits the bones and marrow and is good for any bone pathology. Because it nourishes the blood, it can be

Points	Location	Angles and Depth of Insertion (in)
BL-23 *Shen shu*—bilateral	1.5 *cun* lateral to the lower border of the spinous process of the 2nd lumbar vertebra	Perpendicular. 0.8 – 1.0 ppd. Moxa is applicable
GV-4 *Ming men*	In the depression below the lower border of the spinous process of the 2nd lumbar vertebra	Perpendicular 0.5 – 1.0 ppd. Moxa is applicable
BL-25 *Da chang shu*—bilateral	1.5 *cun* lateral to the lower border of the spinous process of the 4th lumbar vertebra	Perpendicular 0.80 – 1.5 ppd. Moxa is applicable
GV-3 *Yao yang guan*	In the depression below the spinous process of the 4th lumbar vertebra, level with the iliac crest	Perpendicular 0.5 – 1.0 ppd. Moxa is applicable
BL-40 *Wei zhong*—bilateral	At the popliteal crease of the knee, between the tendons of the biceps femoris and semitendinosus muscles	Perpendicular 0.5 – 1.5 ppd or bleed. Moxa is contraindicated (may shorten the tendon)

Table 6.**2** Eight needle technique: points, locations, and angles and depths of insertion

used for anemia, brightening the eyes and alopecia.

The Gate of Life, GV-4 (*ming men*), the original *qi* of the kidney, encompasses kidney *yin* and *yang*, which are inextricably bound together. Therefore, GV-4 is appropriate for the two aspects of kidney *qi* vacuity, that is, kidney *yin* and *yang*. In this capacity it nourishes the original *qi* of preheaven, that is, the person's constitution, basic vitality, and inherited weaknesses on a physical and mental level.

Ming men is the most powerful point to strengthen kidney *yang* and the entire *yang* in general, especially if combined with moxa. It tonifies and warms the "Fire of the Gate of Vitality," resolving kidney *yang* vacuity symptoms such as chilliness, abundant clear urination, diarrhea, and urinary incontinence. *Ming men* fortifies a tired condition and lack of vitality; it alleviates depression, weak knees, and weak legs. A pale tongue and a deep, weak pulse may indicate kidney *yang* vacuity.

Ming men benefits the *yang* aspect of the kidney essence and is indicated in all sexual disorders from weakness of essence evidenced by impotence, premature ejaculation, nocturnal emission, and bone disorders. It strengthens the low back and knees, expels cold, and dries damp-cold, especially with the use of moxa. However, exercise caution with moxa, as it is very warming and can cause heat aggravation, particularly if there are also signs of kidney *yin* vacuity as there may be especially in patients receiving hormonal or radiation therapy for cancer. Discontinue moxa if signs of heat aggravation develop. Other conditions that can be treated include leukorrhea, abdominal, and uterine pain. *Ming men* calms the spirit, benefits and clears the brain. It treats seizures, disorientation, forgetfulness, fear, fright, insomnia, and dizziness.

Da chang shu, BL-25, is the back *shu* point of the large intestine. Remembering the clinical utility of back *shu* points, which are indicated to adjust *qi* and blood, BL-25 eliminates stagnation of *qi* and blood of the intestines that may cause pain, numbness, muscular atrophy, and motor impairment of the back and lower extremities. *Da chang shu* promotes the function of the large intestine and removes obstructions from the channel. It regulates the large intestine and stomach, reducing constipation or diarrhea, dysentery, painful defecation or urination, abdominal distention, and intestinal noise. It benefits low back pain or strain, pain in the sacroiliac joint, and relieves fullness, swelling, and paralysis of the lower extremities.

Yao yang guan, GV-3, tonifies kidney *yang* and *qi*. As such, it strengthens the lower back and legs. It is beneficial for irregular menstruation, nocturnal emission, and impotence. Very frequently used as a local point for backaches, particularly from kidney *yang* vacuity, it is indicated especially when the backache radiates to the legs. It is beneficial for pain in the lumbosacral region, numbness, muscular atrophy, motor impairment, weakness of the legs and knee pain. With moxa it warms cold and dries damp—cold that may produce leukorrhea, diarrhea, colitis, and lower abdominal distention.

Bladder 40 (*wei zhong*) is the *he* (uniting) point of the bladder channel. Elementally, it is the earth point and the controlling point of that channel. As such, it is very effective in clearing and resolving heat and dampness from the bladder and intestines that causes burning urination, ulcerations, diarrhea, and urinary incontinence. It cools the blood and drains heat from the blood especially with a bloodletting technique. Thus, it treats skin diseases, boils, fever, and epistaxis. Lower back pain, sciatica, hip joint pain, restricted movement, lower extremity paralysis, all knee joint diseases, gastrocnemius muscle spasms, convulsions, and muscular tetany can be treated through this point.

As in all cases of tonification and dispersion, needle retention times are relative to the person and will vary. As a general rule however, needles should be retained for approximately 15 to 20 minutes. While the overall effect of the treatment is tonification of kidney *qi* and *yang*, the technique applied to each set of points depends on whether the point needs to be tonified or dispersed. This decision can be made by properly differentiating the patient's condition.

Ten needle technique

In chronic conditions, when vacuity of *qi*, blood, or *yin* is the primary diagnosis, ten needle technique, another treatment strategy I acquired in China, can be used as either a treatment plan in and of itself or as the skeletal formula to which other points may be added based on signs and symptoms. This formula can be applied in a variety of clinical situations. It is obvious in clinical practice that vacuity of the essential substances of *qi*, blood, and *yin* are not only commonly encountered but are difficult to treat because they indicate long-term, chronic conditions. Thus, it is a treatment suitable for cancer patients. Clinically and theoretically this treatment approach is also effective in tonifying *yang* as well. Thus, this formula can address tonifying *qi*, blood, *yin* and yang—certainly an efficient prescription.

Table 6.**3** summarizes the points used in ten needle technique, their locations, and angles and depths of insertion. A discussion of the primary energetics that account for the utility of this valu-

Points	Location	Angles and Depths of Insertion (in)
CV-13 (*shang wan*)	On the midline of the abdomen, 5 *cun* above the center of the umbilicus	0.5–1.2 ppd
CV-12 (*zhong wan*)	On the midline of the abdomen, 4 *cun* above the center of the umbilicus	0.5–1.2 ppd
CV-10 (*xia wan*)	On the midline of the abdomen, 2 *cun* above the center of the umbilicus	0.5–1.2 ppd
ST-25 (*tian shu*)—bilateral	2 *cun* lateral to the center of the umbilicus	0.7–1.2 ppd
ST-36 (*zu san li*)—bilateral	3 *cun* below ST 35, one fingerbreadth lateral to the anterior crest of the tibia	0.5–1.2 ppd
CV-6 (*qi hai*)	On the midline of the abdomen, 1.5 *cun* below the umbilicus	0.8–1.2 ppd
PC-6 (*nei guan*)—bilateral	2 *cun* above the wrist crease, between the tendons of the palmaris longus and flexor carpi radialis muscles	0.5–0.8 ppd

Table 6.**3** Ten needle technique: points, locations, and angles and depths of insertion

able formula follows. A note of caution should be provided concerning the insertion depths of these needles, which are the recommended depths from Chinese texts. As always, these depths are a range and should be adjusted according to the patient's presentation, as many patients are thin, guarded, or vulnerable in the abdominal region and along the conception vessel channel.

CV-13 (*shang guan*) controls the upper orifice of the stomach (cardiac sphincter) so that food can enter the stomach to begin the rottening and ripening process. In this way, food is broken down and *qi*, blood, and *yin* are produced, and stomach *qi* descends more fully. Combined with CV-12 it raises the *yang* and sinking spleen *qi*.

CV-12 (*zhong wan*), the front *mu* point of the stomach, is one of the eight meeting points (*ba hui xue*) that dominates the *fu* organs. As such, it is involved in receiving, digesting, absorbing, transmitting, and transforming food. It regulates stomach *qi* and tonifies chronic spleen and stomach problems such as vacuity of *qi, yin*, or *yang*. It also resolves dampness.

As an important vortex—a crossing point of many channels—CV-12 is a very powerful point. The internal pathway of the lung channel begins at CV-12. The spleen, heart, and small intestine channels pass through *zhong wan*. The liver channel ends there and the large intestine and triple burner channels begin there. The point is located along the *ren* channel pathway. Located at the midpoint of the stomach, it controls the middle of the stomach, tonifying the spleen and stomach so they can produce *qi*, blood, and *yin* and resolve dampness. It regulates stomach *qi* and is useful for chronic stomach and spleen problems. It suppresses rebellious stomach *qi* such as vomiting, and is good for neurasthenia and emotional problems.

CV-10 (*xia guan*) controls the lower orifice of the stomach (pylorus), encouraging stomach *qi* to descend. It relieves food stagnation and tonifies the spleen and stomach so that food is broken down and transformed into *qi*, blood, or *yin*. Due to its lower location in relation to the stomach, it is helpful in indigestion, stomach ache, and prolapse of the stomach, diarrhea, and acute stomach problems.

ST-25 (*tian shu*), as the front *mu* point of the large intestine, according to the ancient *Huang Di Nei Jing* text, adjusts the intestines in any condition, that is, it clears heat, regulates *qi*, relieves food retention, and eliminates stagnation. According to the *Nan Jing, The Classic of Difficult Issues*, Stomach 25 is the front *mu* point of the lungs so the lungs can be treated specifically at ST-25 on the right side of the body.

On the left side, ST-25 can treat blood stagnation and liver blood stagnation in particular. The reason for this is that at the site of ST-25 on the left, the portal vein, which carries nutrients to the liver to be packaged into packets of glycogen or stored energy, exits from the large intestine and goes to the liver. As a result, when liver *qi* is stagnant, it frequently leads to liver blood stagnation and manifests at ST-25 on the left because of this liver–large intestine connection. Correspondingly, when there is a blockage at Stomach 25 on the left, it can cause liver *qi* stagnation. When this point is not blocked and is free-flowing, it opens the lower burner and the channels to nourish the *qi* of the lower burner. It is a storehouse of energy.

ST-36 (*zu san li*) opens the lower burner, regulates the intestines, and builds kidney *yin*. It brings energy down. It benefits and regulates the stomach and spleen, controlling the epigastric area. As the lower *he* (uniting) point, ST-36 sends a vessel directly to the stomach. As the horary point on an earth channel, ST-36 tonifies and adjusts the *qi* and blood of the whole body. It stimulates *qi* production and dispels cold. It strengthens the body's resistance, increases immunity, and strengthens the anti-pathogenic factor. It regulates *yin* and *wei qi* (defense *qi*). It raises the *yang* and strengthens weak and vacuous conditions.

CV-6 (*qi hai*) is at the center of the vital energy in the body, the *dan tian*, where the living *qi* of the kidney resides. It is useful for all states of exhaustion and insufficiency. Especially with the use of moxa, it tonifies *qi, yang* and *yin*, regulates *qi*, tonifies original *qi*, resolves damp and augments kidney vacuity.

PC-6 (*nei guan*) assists in communication between, and treatment of, the three burners; it keeps *qi* and blood flowing in their proper pathway. As master of the *yin wei mai* (*yang* linking vessel) it produces *yin* defensive energy. Coupled with the spleen channel and the *chong mai* PC-6 assists spleen and kidney functions.

It is apparent from an analysis of this formula that ten needle technique is a beneficial formula to employ when there is a multiplicity of symptoms pointing in the direction of vacuity, a condition cancer patients exhibit. Sometimes very vacuous patients whom this formula would benefit cannot tolerate the insertion of ten needles, in which case the following modifications can be made:

1. Needle PC-6 (*nei guan*) only on the left side because pericardium energetics are more left-sided as evidenced by the pulse system.
2. Pretest by palpation CV-13 (*shang wan*), CV-12 (*zhong wan*), and CV-10 (*xia wan*), and select the tenderest point to needle instead of all three.
3. As "Heaven's Pivot," ST-25 (*tian tu*) should always be needled bilaterally to establish equilibrium between *qi* and blood. As was discussed previously under the energetics of that point, ST-25 on the right side is a *qi* reflex point and ST-25 on the left is a blood stagnation point. Needling both points helps to balance *qi* and blood.
4. CV-6 (*qi hai*) should always be included in this strategy.
5. ST-36 (*zu san li*) can be needled only on the right side due to the affinity of stomach energetics for the right side, again as depicted in the pulse system.

This modification can be effective especially if the practitioner's tonification needle technique is proficient enough to compensate for the reduced number of needles. If no signs of heat are present, either of the excess or vacuity type, the addition of moxa is incomparable, particularly for tonifying the *yang*.

After the administration of the ten needle technique, patients will not experience a great surge of energy but rather a deep-seated feeling of relaxation and perhaps even tiredness as the energy being tonified consolidates itself on a very deep level. Patients should be advised of this therapeutic reaction so they know what to expect. This plan can be administered as a course of treatment, that is, ten consecutive treatments or as a periodic tonification treatment.

Chinese Immunity Formula

At Guananmen Hospital, the largest cancer hospital in Beijing where an integrative Chinese/Western approach is employed to treat cancer patients, the Chinese doctors I studied with proposed acupuncture treatment to assist patients in recovery from cancer. As a result of standard Western treatments for cancer, these patients generally have a weakened immune response, as Yan et al. confirm: "The cellular immune response is usually impaired in cancer patients, and especially in those with advanced disease. This is further compromised by radiation and/or chemotherapy."[20] Nagano also agrees when he points out that "Cancer patients are susceptible to infections due to an underactive immune system, malnutrition, radiation or drugs used in therapy that are partly responsible."[21] Table 6.**4** can be consulted for the points in this prescriptions and their contribution to the immune enhancement for cancer patients.

The dual purpose of this strategy is 1) to combat the side-effects of chemotherapy, surgery, radiation, and other medications and procedures and 2) to support the anti-pathogenic *qi*. This point prescription provides potent tonification of the body. It can be modified based upon the patient's presentation with points deleted or added according to signs and symptoms. A tonification needle technique should be used.

Needles are inserted to the standard Chinese angles and depths of insertion. A gentle needle technique in terms of *de qi* sensation is preferable. Needles may be retained for up to 20 minutes. Patients may be treated daily if this is feasible. Mild, indirect moxibustion may be applied to all points, however, carefully monitor signs and symptoms of heat aggravation since *yin* vacuity with heat is a common sequel to Western treatment.

Selected Point Categories

Keeping all the principles discussed in this chapter in mind, we must also remember to treat what we see. The following categories of points have been found to be clinically effective in the treatment of cancer.[23] An example of liver cancer is provided to illustrate the use of the points:

1. *Xi* (cleft) points of the channel for corresponding organ pain, i. e., LR-6 (*zhong du*) for pain in the liver area, the primary Chinese treatment strategy for cancerous pain.
2. A combination of the paired *mu/shu* points for organs and weak constitution, i. e., BL-18 (*gan shu*), LR-14 (*qi men*).

Points	Functions
ST-36 (*zu san li*)	Brings energy down, especially rebellious stomach *qi* that is a common sequel to chemotherapy or radiation. Prevents vomiting and loss of body fluids necessary to re-establish post-natal *qi*. Tonifies stomach and kidney *yin* damaged by Western treatment. Increases white blood cell count markedly.* Increases T-lymphocytes in elderly with indirect moxa every other day for 10 minutes
PC-6 (*nei guan*)	As master of the *yin wei* channel, tonifies *yin* defensive energy. Brings energy down, quiets the heart, soothes the emotions, quells the nausea that may accompany chemotherapy
LI-4 (*he gu*)	Stops pain, brings the energy down for nausea due to chemotherapy. Increases phagocytic reaction
SP-6 (*san yin jiao*)	Group *luo* of the three-leg *yin*; tonifies *yin* of liver, spleen, and kidney, whose *yin* is damaged by treatment such as radiation
CV-12 (*zhong wan*)	As front *mu* point of the stomach, tonifies stomach *yin*. Brings down rebellious stomach *qi*. Reinforces the spleen and strengthens the kidney
HT-7 (*shen men*)	As the earth point and sedation point on the heart channel, it levels the heart, calms the spirit, and makes pain negligible. A primary point for pain

*Meng, 1992, see References, note 22.

Table 6.**4** Analysis of point function in the Chinese treatment of immunity

3. Proximal/distal points on the channel pathway to alleviate pain, i. e., LR-4 (*zhong feng*), LR-8 (*qu quan*).
4. Lower *he* (uniting) points for cancer of the corresponding organs, i. e., LR-8 (*qu quan*).
5. Points that treat the heart and liver because of their relationship to *qi* and blood, i. e., LR-4 (*zhong feng*), HT-7 (*shen men*).
6. Confluent (master and coupled points of the eight extraordinary vessels) and influential points because of the domains that they govern.

Moxa: Treat the Root

Studies have shown the clinical utility of employing moxibustion for energetically increasing the *yang* of the body, emotionally increasing the will, and physically raising the white blood cell count. The effects of moxibustion are useful, in fact, prerequisite for all cases of vacuity be it in general, or specific subsets of the population such as the elderly or patients who are immunocompromised as long as there are no heat manifestations. (See examples of moxa application provided in this chapter.)

Conclusion

Western medicine's treatment of cancer is, no doubt, severe. Its side-effects alone are myriad and debilitating. However, we must never lose sight of the fact that the treatment of cancer by Western medicine saves lives. By contrast, each integrated TCM approach to dealing with cancer and/or the side-effects of Western drugs or radiation treatments has a major focus on generally improving the overall constitution of the patient. The aim of integrated treatment plans is manifold. Among its goals and benefits are:

- to afford the patient a better quality of life during and after Western medical treatments for cancer;
- to strengthen the body such that the patient can complete the recommended Western course of treatment;
- to treat the root, or *yin/yang* imbalance that was instrumental in the creation of the cancer; and
- to aid in the prevention of recurrence or metastases of the cancer.

It can be successful within limits with many of these factors. The treatment of cancer is indeed formidable, but one we can embrace because we are empowered with two of the greatest medical systems in the world. The challenge is to energetically and compassionately employ them equally.

References

1. Curties D. *Massage Therapy & Cancer*. New Brunswick: Curties-Overzet Publications; 1999:8.
2. Op. Cit.:10 – 11.
3. Pan MJ. *Cancer Treatment with Fu Zheng Pei Ben Principle*. Fujian: China Fujian Science and Technology Publishing House; 1992:2 – 8, 18.
4. Zhang DZ. *The Treatment of Cancer by Integrated Chinese-Western Medicine*. Zhang Ting-liang, Flaws B, trans. Boulder, CO: Blue Poppy Press; 1989:21 – 22.
5. Zhao RJ. Paradoxes in cancer treatment—and the light in this black hole. *Tra Chi Med World* April 2000;(2):8, 9, 30 – 31.
6. See 4, p. 130.
7. See 4, p. 138.
8. Gelles W. Qi. *J Tra Eastern Health and Fitness*. Winter 1993:12.
9. See 3, p. 37.
10. Maciocia G. *The Practice of Chinese Medicine*. London: Churchill Livingstone, Inc; 1994:438.
11. Hsu HY. *Treating Cancer with Chinese Herbs*. Long Beach, California: Oriental Healing Arts Institute; 1982:3.
12. Cheung CS. *Strategies in the Management of Cancer—a Series of Works by Chinese Scholars*. San Francisco, California: Harmonious Sunshine Cultural Center; 1993.
13. See 3, p. 37.
14. See 3, p. 38.
15. See 3, p. 37 – 39.
16. See 4, p. 94.
17. See 4, p. 64, 92.
18. See 3, p. 47– 48.
19. See 1, p. 24.
20. Yan S, Hersh E, Lee SL, Wong W, Loo TL, Mavlight GM. Immune restoration and/or augmentation of local graft versus host reaction by traditional Chinese medicinal herbs. *Inter J O Med*. 1984;1(1):41.
21. Nagano K. Immune enhancement through acupuncture and moxibustion; specific treatment for allergic disorders, mild infectious disease and secondary infection. *Amer J Acu* 1991;19(4): 331.
22. Meng C. Current status of research abroad concerning the effect of acupuncture and moxibustion on immunologic functions. *J Tra Chi Med*. 1992;12(3):212.
23. Fu WB, Zhang B. Contemplation of the treatment of cancer pain by acupuncture. *TCM Shanghai J Acu and Moxi*. 2000 English ed. 3rd issue:57 – 60.

7 Geriatric Disorders: Clinical Considerations and Treatment Modalities in Working with Elderly Patients in an Institutional Setting

Working with elderly patients in a nursing home or similar institutional environment is a challenging task for a practitioner of any discipline. Although individually the number of illnesses these patients may suffer from is quite large, as a group they share certain conditions in common, which distinguish them from other patients receiving Oriental medical treatment. The practitioner needs to become aware of these features in order to deliver the best healthcare possible to this sometimes neglected segment of our population.

While treatment modalities are almost intrinsically connected to diagnosis, there are still general treatment principles that are part of the infrastructure of Oriental medicine that are worthy options for this group of patients. If the practitioner has an opportunity to treat such patients he/she should realize that geriatric patients are different from the average person encountered in an outpatient setting. Because of their age, delicate condition, and clinical complexity, there are treatment adaptations that are critical in the care of the elderly person.

Additionally, a more generalized diagnostic approach to thinking about the older patient is presented, such as the complexity of their medical history, possible drug and herbal interactions, how to diagnose their pain, and classical and modern Oriental approaches to aging, which can illuminate treatment plans, acupuncture points, and herbal selection. Each of these parameters is discussed below.

The problems of the elderly are frequently compound and complex. Their problems can range from physical to mental, and some may have both. This is no surprise to the practitioner who sees the relationship between the physical and mental manifestations of the self. There is a preponderance of mental disorders such as senile dementia or Alzheimer's disease and from a Chinese perspective, there can be complicated syndromes characterized by the secondary pathological products of stagnant blood and phlegm, which are pernicious and difficult to treat. Patients in nursing homes, assisted living centers or other similar environments are also confined due to a variety of reasons. Whether ambulatory, bedridden or wheelchair-bound, in general they require a degree of care they or their family cannot provide.

In directing treatment toward the elderly, combine compassion with realism. Consider their conditions to see what you can do. To a certain degree some of their symptoms can be addressed. Aid and comfort in the form of human interaction, appropriate professional touch, and the instruments of Oriental medicine, can go a long way, so while cure may not be attainable, the reconciliation of the condition, that is, healing, can occur. The specific guidelines for treatment that I have used to direct my treatment approach for the elderly are discussed below.

■ General Guidelines for the Treatment of Patients in Institutional Settings

1. Make sure you have the written consent of your patient or appropriate guardian when treating the elderly patient.
2. With all patients, medical history is important, but thorough personal medical history is of utmost importance in treating the elderly due to their often weakened condition and the multiple illnesses they may have. Obtain a complete medical history so you know all the conditions the patient has. It is more likely that they have a more lengthy medical history than a younger person simply due to age. You will probably need to get this information from the patient's medical chart as they may not remember their

complete history or have the ability to talk at length with you. Due to the patient's age, length of the history, memory problems, and complexity of the case, communication with their physician is important. Hence. the Oriental medical provider should cultivate skills in communicating with the Western doctor. Diagnosed illnesses will usually imply that the patients are also taking multiple Western medications, which singularly or in combination may produce certain side-effects, which can be further complicated with Oriental herbs. See a discussion of herbs and the elderly later in this chapter.
3. Discuss anything in the medical chart you don't understand with the patient's assigned medical personnel such as their doctor or nurse.
4. Treat those who are able to articulate how they feel or those you feel can sustain and benefit from Oriental medical therapy.
5. When you have identified the complaint against the background of their medical history, explain to the patient and/or their family in clear, simple terms what you will be doing, what you hope to attain, what techniques you will be using, and what the treatments may feel like. Don't make promises about the outcome, but do inform each group about all of these things so they have a sense about what is occurring in treatment and its possible outcome.
6. Proceed slowly. Do not attempt to do too much in any one treatment, especially for the elderly whose vital *qi* is weak. Evaluate therapeutic outcome weekly.
7. Patients are individuals. Choose the modality of treatment that best corresponds to the patient's condition. The major modalities employed in Oriental medicine for the elderly and their suitability are discussed later and summarized at the end of this chapter in Table 7.**5**.
8. Realize that for the most part, these patients are now in their final home. They are here to be cared for. This is probably the place where they will die and many of them know this. They may be despondent and depressed. While the things you can do for them may be limited, your presence alone can give them solace and that attention is good medicine.

Treatment Adaptations

Patient Positioning

As with the administration of most acupuncture, a supine position is generally recommended for treatment. Especially with the elderly though, there are times when this is not possible due to their limitations. However, if a treatment must be administered in a sitting position such as in bed or a wheelchair use caution in needling chest points such as LU-1 (*zhong fu*) or CV-17 (*shan zhong*). In general, avoid abdominal needling such as CV-12 (*zhong wan*) in such patients. In these cases, if the patient moves in treatment or has a sagging posture, the needle could become displaced and possibly cause a pneumothorax, break, bend, or become deeply embedded in the tissues.

Be careful treating patients reclining on their stomachs when receiving acupuncture. Support their necks with a face cradle that is properly angled. This position may be contraindicated for patients with respiratory illnesses, back pain, severe abdominal distention or illnesses of the abdominal cavity, or for patients on oxygen.

Geriatric Pathology: Kidney Vacuity, Stagnant Blood, and Phlegm

Historically in Chinese medicine, most illnesses of the elderly have been attributed to the decline of kidney *qi* as outlined in the *qi* cycles for men and women (see Figs 7.**1** and 7.**2**), or a combination of spleen and kidney vacuity. While kidney *qi*, which is responsible for growth, maturation, and development, inevitably declines over time, the illnesses of the elderly should be relatively benign if we use this model exclusively to predict aging pathology. Under this scenario hearing diminishes, teeth and bones become brittle, hair grays or is lost, the menses cease, eyesight lessens, and digestive disorders ensue. Certainly these conditions do indeed occur, yet as physicians we know that the illnesses most of the elderly are developing today are much more complex, devastating, and life-threatening than those one would predict according to the kidney *qi*.

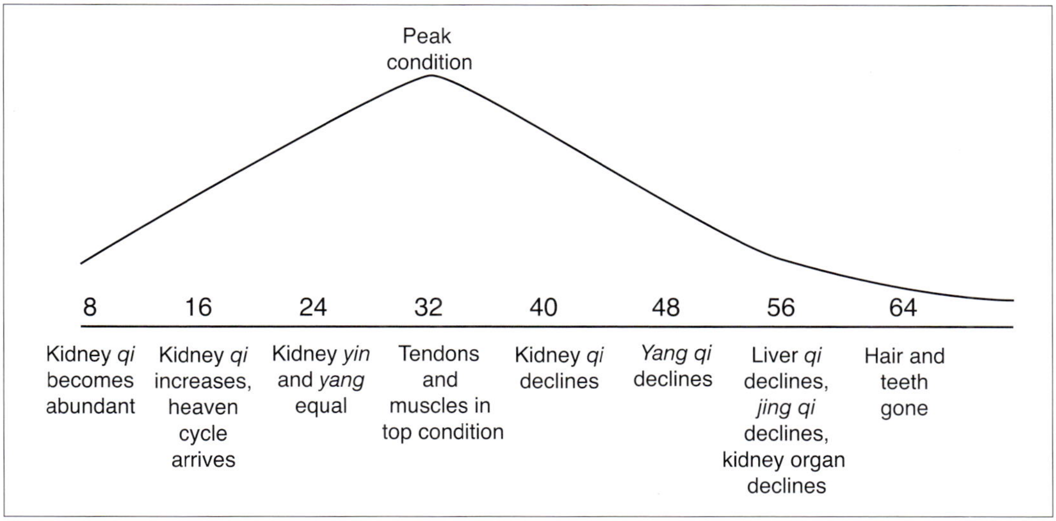

Fig. 7.**1** The *qi* cycle for men.

Age 8 The kidney *qi* becomes abundant, the hair begins to grow longer, and the teeth begin to change.

Age 16 The kidney *qi* becomes more abundant, he begins to have his heaven cycle, he is full of *jing-qi* (semen), he can ejaculate and have a child; intercourse (*yin/yang* harmonization possible).

Age 24 The kidney *qi* is equal (i.e., kidney *yin/yang* are balanced), the tendons, muscles, bones, become strong; the wisdom teeth grow.

Age 32 All tendons, muscles, bones in top condition.

Age 40 The kidney *qi* weakens, the hair begins to fall off, and the teeth begin to wither.

Age 48 The *yang qi* in the upper part of the body declines, with the complexion looking withered, hair turns grey.

Age 56 The liver *qi* begins to weaken, the heaven cycle becomes exhausted, the *jing-qi* (semen) becomes scanty, and the kidney organs decline, and all parts of the body begin to grow old.

Age 64 All hair and teeth are gone.

Stagnant Blood

Yan De-Xin, a contemporary Chinese physician, has revolutionized Chinese views on gerontology with his thesis that most modern day illnesses are caused by blood stagnation. It is his theory that static blood (*yu xue*), a causative factor of illness in and of itself, likewise is the etiological precursor, which can cause multiple *qi* and blood disorders.

In Chinese medical theory, blood stagnation is problematic because it involves blood and *qi* stasis, and movement of both are requisite for the healthy human organism. This physiological occurrence seems to be an integral part of the pathologies of aging, and the reader, if interested, should acquaint him/herself with Yan De-Xin's thesis, which expounds the etiology and subtle clinical manifestations of blood stagnation.[1] Table 7.**1** shows the patterns of static blood as gleaned from subjective symptoms, medical history, physical exam, organ systems, and laboratory findings, according to Yan De-Xin[2], and a diagnosis of static blood pattern may made by looking at the evidence of all these things. Clinically, if there are more than four criteria within any two of these categories, one may diagnose the disease as manifesting a pattern of static blood.

Yan De-Xin amply supports his theory with classical sources. One idea he advances is that drugs are a leading cause of blood stagnation. Because the elderly may be on or may have taken many drugs, their health is intimately connected to their drug history. His preventative regimes revolve around strengthening the *qi*, activating the blood, and transforming stasis. For the clinician, this suggests the use of blood-activating herbs and acupuncture points, which perform similar functions. Consult "Recognition and prevention of herb–drug interactions" by Chen[3] to ascertain that the blood stasis herbs chosen are not contraindicated for the patient, for instance that the patient

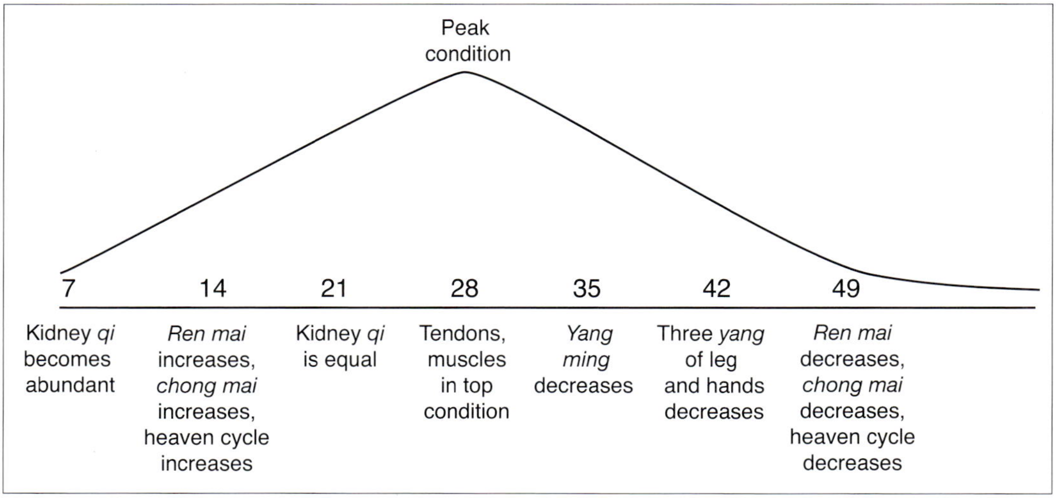

Fig. 7.**2** The *qi* cycle for women.
Age 7 The kidney *qi* becomes abundant, the hair begins to grow longer, and the teeth begin to change.
Age 14 The *ren mai* begins to flow, the heaven cycle begins, and the *chong mai* begins to grow in abundance, menstruation begins, pregnancy is possible.
Age 21 The kidney *qi* becomes equal (i.e., the *yin/yang* are balanced), the wisdom teeth begin to grow.
Age 28 The tendons, muscles, bones become hard, the hair grows to the longest, the body and mind are in top condition.
Age 35 The *yang ming* channels begin to weaken with the result that the complexion starts to wither, the hair begins to fall off.
Age 42 The three *yang* channels of the hands and legs begin to weaken, the complexion looks even more withered, the hair turns grey.
Age 49 The *ren mai* becomes deficient, the heaven cycle becomes exhausted, the *chong mai* becomes weakened and scanty, her body becomes old, she can not become pregnant

is not on Coumadin (warfarin—a blood thinner) or has any coagulation problems.

Acupuncture does not have the biological complexity of herbs because the needles regulate the physiological functioning of *qi* and blood. Table 7.**2** provides a prioritized list of the points I have found to be the most useful in activating the blood. I highly recommend the integration of at least one of these into any acupuncture prescription. If not actually needled they can be palpated by the practitioner prior to treatment as part of a diagnostic assessment of blood stagnation. Additionally, the patient can be taught to stimulate these points on a daily basis by rubbing them vigorously for two to three seconds or the practitioner may do so during treatment. If needling is performed, needles may be inserted to the standard depths of insertion in the standard locations using a dispersion technique. Needling retention time depends upon the balance of the treatment the practitioner is administering but is usually 10–15 minutes.

Phlegm

Contemporary and ancient scholars provide added insight into geriatric pathology in their discussions of the secondary pathological product of phlegm. Of course, in Oriental medicine the concept of phlegm is very complex and extends beyond the narrow definition of respiratory secretions, but those well trained in Oriental medicine should understand its nuances. Some interesting concepts about phlegm from Cheung[4] are listed below and can be applied to the elderly. Following each of these scholarly observations, I have listed my comments in parentheses:

1. *To manage intractable diseases and bizarre disorders never overlook the possibility of phlegm.* (Certainly many geriatric diseases such as Alzheimer's are intractable and bizarre and seem to have a phlegm component.)
2. *When definitive management fails the hidden culprit may be phlegm.* (It is difficult to manage

Signs and Symptoms of Static Blood	
Subjective symptoms	
Fever	Generalized fever, for instance, tidal fever. Local fever in specific areas, i.e., skin, muscle, etc.
Pain	Immovable, fixed
Bleeding	Excessive and difficult to stop as in hemoptysis, hemafecia
Distention	Certain areas of the body such as head and eyes experience distention that does not decrease. Continues over time
Itching	Feeling of crawling beneath skin
Numbness	Inability to feel or electrical feeling, lack of perception of heat and cold
Stiffness	Stiff, inhibited movement such as with the neck
Dry mouth	Mouth dry, but not thirsty
Dreams	Little sleep but dreams of danger and fright
Memory	Insomnia, palpitations, poor memory
Mental states	Senility, dementia, crazy speech
Symptoms in the organ systems	
Heart	Palpitations, heart pain, disturbed *shen*, mania, angina
Liver/ Gall bladder	Depression, agitation, easy vesation, floaters
Spleen/ Stomach	Epigastric and abdominal pain and aching, lack of eating, constipation, diarrhea
Lung	Enduring cough, panting, phlegm tinged with blood
Kidney	Lower abdominal distention, urination problems, constipation
Physical signs	
Hair	Withered, dry, yellowish, weak hair
Face	Dark complexion
Eyes	Dark around the orbit, yellow sclera
Ears	Deafness
Cheeks	Red flush or lines
Nose	Red marks
Lips	Dark lips
Chin	Dark chin
Tongue	Dark red or purple with stasis marks
Neck	Distended veins, lumps
Chest	Stirring or throbbing of chest
Abdomen	Abdominal distention, masses, hardness
Back	Painful protruding vertebrae
Limbs	Enlarged toes and fingers, coldness
Skin	Stiff dry scaly skin, lumps, moles, patches
Voice	Hoarseness
History	
Chronic illness	Enduring disease must have stasis
Surgery	Internal adhesions and scars
Menses	Menstrual problems
Reproduction	Infertility, menopause
Lifestyle	Smoking, alcohol, sweet, fatty foods
Injury	External
Laboratory examination	
Blood	Viscosity of blood and plasma increased, hyperlipidemia, high bilirubin, increased erythrocytes, leukocytes, and platelets
Nail bed circulation	Increased capillary loops, decreased velocity, exudation, and bleeding
Cardiac system	Damaged myocardium, enlarged heart, diseased valves, reduced blood flow
Internal organs	Enlarged spleen and liver, lung or abdominal tumors, polyps, diverticula
Brain	Cerebral arteriosclerosis, epilepsy, cerebral hematoma or tumor

Table 7.**1** Patterns of static blood

Points	Energetics
KI-1 (*yong quan*)	The primary point for vascular problems. Diagnostic and treatment point for blood disturbances anywhere in the body. Improves circulation and regulates blood pressure because the source of blood is in the kidneys
LI-4 (*he gu*)	As the metal point on a wood channel (metal controls wood), regulates the smooth flow of *qi* in the lower burner. Because the blood follows the *qi*, it regulates blood flow as well. Major point to move blood stagnation in lower *jiao* (one of the three burners)
SP-10 (*xue hai*)	Sea of Blood point. Intersects with the *chong mai* vessel. Treats blood stagnation anywhere in the body, particularly in the lower abdomen
BL-17 (*ge shu*)	Influential point that dominates the blood. Back *shu* point of the diaphragm. Moves the blood by moving the *qi* of the diaphragm
ST-25 L (*tian shu*)	Diagnostic point for blood stagnation anywhere in the body due to its connection to the liver. At this point, the portal vein goes to the liver
SP-6 (*san yin jiao*)	For blood stagnation in the abdomen due to poor venous circulation or problems of the liver, spleen, and kidney channels in bringing *qi* and blood to the middle *jiao*

Table 7.**2** Clinically effective points to resolve blood stasis

many geriatric diseases, hence phlegm is likely involved.)

3. *Dysfunction of every organ can generate phlegm.* (As we know, with age, organ function declines; hence the possibility of phlegm formation escalates.)
4. *Eight out of ten people are plagued by phlegm.* (Apart from obvious clinical manifestations, statistically the elderly are automatically part of this group.)
5. *Prolonged retention of turbid phlegm will easily cause an accumulation of static retention of ecchymotic blood, which will promote congealing of phlegm.* (This illustrates the cyclic inter-relationship between phlegm and blood stasis. Phlegm can lead to blood stasis, which in turn can exacerbate the original problem of phlegm. Additionally, blood and phlegm have the same origin, which is fluid. Hence, there is often a common denominator between the origins of static blood and phlegm formation.)
6. *In terms of treatment many ancient scholars admonish, "Those who are skillful in managing phlegm, do not directly treat phlegm, but treat qi."* (Treating the *qi* certainly assists the practitioner in addressing the root of the problem to bring about greater resolution of the phlegm. As we have already established, *qi* vacuity is also a major component in illnesses due the natural decline of vital *qi*. As far as an overall treatment strategy is concerned this approach makes sense, because it is the vacuity of the organs' functions that is the root of the phlegm formation.)

Phlegm is a difficult pathology to remediate because its nature is heavy, turbid, and sticky, and its formation is usually a result of *zang fu* organ dysfunction, static blood, or pre-existing phlegm. In the elderly, diseases characterized by phlegm are numerous. They include gallstones and kidney stones, atherosclerotic plaques, arthritic bone deformities, mania, psychosis, memory problems, edema, facial paralysis, cough, chronic bronchitis, joint pain, stroke, digestive disorders, angina, vertigo, coma, burning leg sensations, and atrophic limbs. For perhaps the most comprehensive discussion of phlegm see CS Cheung's *Abstract and Clinical Review* article on phlegm[4], which details it in its myriad formations with corresponding differentiations and herbal formulae. Table 7.**3** reminds the practitioner of points that are clinically effective in the resolution of phlegm. It comprises the points I have found most useful in its management.

Points	Energetics
LI-14 (*bi nao*)	Resolves phlegm and disperses masses anywhere in the body, particularly in the upper *jiao* and head
ST-40 (*feng long*)	As the *luo* point of the stomach, sweeps phlegm from the body
SP-4 (*gong sun*)	Drains excesses such as damp and phlegm from the spleen and stomach
CV-12 (*zhong wan*)	Resolves phlegm in the spleen and stomach

Table 7.**3** Clinically effective points to resolve phlegm

Physical Limitations

As they age, some patients will never regain full control over their bodies. Like them, we need to recognize these physical limitations. For instance, do not try to make a patient walk without a walker if the patient's physician has required it or if the patient is incapable of walking. Likewise, check bone density levels in suspect patients to see if they have the weight-bearing capacity to allow them to walk. Ultimately, what we are trying to do in our treatment is to enhance the quality of life of the patient. Oriental medicine can assist in this goal because it is predicated on natural forces that promote proper physiological functioning.

Pain

Many of the disorders suffered by the elderly have pain as a component, and this pain is usually chronic. As such, it tends to affect the quality of life adversely. Whether it is the pain of an illness like arthritis, or low back pain, chronic neuropathy, advanced painful malignancies, post-fracture or post-operative pain, pain relief should be part of a larger pain management plan that usually requires several modalities. Appropriate treatment plans require a precise differentiation of the pain. A comprehensive discussion of pain differentiation and a multi-disciplinary pain management plan is listed in my article "The differential diagnosis of pain in classical Chinese medicine."[5]

While an Oriental medical practitioner's frame of reference for treating pain is very broad due to its definition of pain, the Western model has more limitations. Even the National Institute of Health's *Consensus Statement* maintains that acupuncture, *tai qi*, *qi gong*, and *tuina* techniques adapted for the elderly are useful therapies; there are few side-effects—a consideration of note, especially for a population that has many health disorders.[6]

Treatment Modalities

The TDP Lamp or the Mineral Infrared Therapy Device

The TDP lamp or the far infrared device are two superb tools for conferring therapeutic heat that can correct many conditions. Due to the size of the lamp they are not the most practical tools to bring to a nursing home on every trip, but if they can be stored there they are excellent choices for elderly patients. The heat of the lamp is relaxing, soothing, and comforting. The modality itself is non-invasive and able to treat large local areas such as the back or abdomen. The use of the lamp is suitable for a variety of conditions, especially *yang* vacuity that the elderly tend towards, by promoting increased metabolism and increased blood circulation.

Excellent results can be obtained both for musculoskeletal problems such as shoulder, back, or neck tension, or for internal problems such as frequent night-time urination, diabetes, insomnia, skin disorders, and neurasthenia. The lamp is effective for other problems such as arthritis, soft tissue injuries, sciatica, bedsores, or the rehabilitation and restoration of any diminished normal function following illness, injury, surgical intervention, or age-related degeneration. As with any treatment, frequency of treatment and length of application of the therapy vary according to the patient's presentation.

A generalization for most conditions would be to treat with the lamp once a week for 10 minutes. Because the elderly may have decreased neurological functioning or diminished sensitivity to heat, which inhibits their ability to report the temperature to you, do not leave them unattended. Stay with them and monitor the skin temperature about every 5 minutes to be sure that the skin is not too hot or burning.

Each of the devices works slightly differently and more can be read about each particular device by consulting the product literature but what they have in common are all of the aforementioned features. See Chapter 20 for a further discussion of the TDP lamp and Figure 20.**1** for a photograph.

Palpation

Palpation is the process of examining the surface of the body by touch to detect the presence of disease. Sometimes it involves the use of pressure to certain points or areas to determine the patient's reaction to that touch. This technique is usually not that effective if the patient's vitality is low as is the case for many of the elderly. They tend not to be able to respond to the diagnostic palpation. Patients may also perceive the procedure as painful instead of as a message about their bodily condition. However, areas of heat, cold, tension, or flaccidity can be determined through palpation and interpreted by the practitioner. Be gentle.

Scalp Acupuncture

Scalp acupuncture is a microsystem of Oriental medicine, which utilizes needling points on the scalp to treat a variety of disorders. It is highly effective for a subset of conditions such as musculoskeletal problems that include muscular atrophy, motor impairment, sequelae of post-stroke disorders, paralysis, involuntary movement problems, multiple sclerosis, and other difficult-to-treat conditions where there is nervous system involvement. The elderly in nursing homes may have many of these ailments.

Electricity

Electrical acupuncture is a method by which electricity is applied to acupuncture needles in order to provoke a constant stimulus to the needles, which is difficult and even impossible to achieve by hand, or to impart an electrical charge to an acupuncture point. It can be employed for numerous conditions, most notably *bi*-syndromes, which are conditions characterized by obstruction with symptoms of pain, or inflammation. Electricity is useful in inducing analgesia because of its superior ability to stimulate the needles with a frequency that cannot be elicited by hand. It is the frequency of stimulation that disperses the obstruction causing the pain or inflammation.

Personally, I do not employ electricity to any patient due to its cold nature. Additionally, because many symptoms of the elderly can be categorized as *yang* vacuity, it may be incompatible with their conditions. The stimulus can also be very jarring and unpleasant, particularly to a delicate older person. The use of electricity is contraindicated for patients with heart conditions and pacemakers.

Needles

Needles of course are the primary instrument of Oriental medicine. They are used to regulate the flow of *qi* and blood in the channels. Needles may be employed to treat the elderly, however, keep the following points in mind when treating these patients:

- Their vital *qi* may be weak, hence it becomes difficult to get the *de qi* stimulus.
- Due to decreased vital *qi*, use few needles so as not to deplete the patient's energy. In general, apply a mild stimulus if any and insert shallowly.
- All body parts may not be readily accessible to needling if the patient is in a wheelchair or bedridden so select points in consideration of the patient's ability to move. Through the microsystem of the ear or the scalp however, all body parts and organs can be treated with needles. Both are excellent choices.
- Fine needles inserted with a tube should be used to prevent bruising, bleeding, or trauma to these delicate patients. I recommend using a #1 gauge, 30 mm Seirin needle.

Point	Energetics
1. *Shen men*	Quiets the heart, calms the spirit, and puts the patient into a state of receptivity for the treatment. For restlessness and common mental disorders. Neutralizes toxins, cures inflammation. Additionally is one of the best clinically effective points for pain because it pertains to the heart. The *Huang Di Nei Jing* text says, "When the Heart is serene, all pain is negligible." Good for insomnia. The elderly may have all of these as problems
2. Sympathetic (three locations)	Relieves pain. The elderly have many disorders characterized by pain. Regulates the autonomic nervous system. Dilates blood vessels; for opthamalogical diseases
3. Kidney	To tonify the root *qi* of the body, the foundation *yin* and *yang*, which declines with aging
4–5. Spleen and stomach	To reinforce post-natal *qi*, which is frequently weak in the elderly due to age and poor nutrition. Builds blood. Since the spleen dominates the muscles, this combination is good for weak muscles that the elderly may have due to lack of exercise or other factors
6. Brain	Regulates neurological function, benefits the mind. Regulates excitation or inhibition of the cerebral cortex. General treatment point for diseases of the nervous, digestive, endocrine, and urogenital systems. For neuropsychiatric disorders. Also for insomnia and prolapse, common in the elderly
7. Liver	Promotes free-flowingness of *qi* in the body. Maintains the harmonious relationship between the internal and external environment. Moves blood, moves stagnation, builds blood and *yin*, increases energy

Note: Modify according to other signs and symptoms; i.e., add points for specific conditions or areas of pain such as prostate, low back, or hypertension.

Table 7.**4** Standardized ear treatment for geriatric patients

Auricular acupuncture

Auricular acupuncture is a method of diagnosing and treating through the microsystem of the ear. It is one of the most useful methods of treatment for any patient regardless of age or condition. It has a high rate of efficacy in adjusting the flow of *qi* and blood in a relatively non-invasive manner, and is suitable for musculoskeletal, internal, emotional, chronic, and acute problems including pain and inflammation. The ear is easily accessible to treat.

Auricular acupuncture is an extremely effective modality to employ for the elderly; in fact, it is my method of choice. Table 7.**4** presents a core ear acupuncture treatment I have constructed, which I use as a skeletal outline in the treatment of elderly patients. Based upon specific signs and symptoms, this formula may be modified. An illustration of these points is also provided in Figure 7.**3**.

Almost unequivocally I employ gold Magrain pellets in one ear then alternate ears for subsequent treatments. Clean the ear well. Use gold pellets to ward off infection in patients who may have reduced wound-healing capacity. Retain the pellets for 3 to 5 days unless the patient is exposed to water or high humidity levels, which could increase the risk of infection—in which case the pellets are worn for fewer days. Instruct the patient to stimulate the pellet mildly for 3 to 5 seconds about 3 to 5 times a day or see if an attendant or family member can do so. The ear is an extremely powerful vortex of energy, yet auricular acupuncture is relatively gentle, well accepted, easy to learn and administer. Remember to remove or provide written instructions for the patient or the caregiver to remove the pellets within 3 to 5 days to guard against infection or if the pellet becomes uncomfortable to the patient, or plan to return to the nursing home to do this yourself.

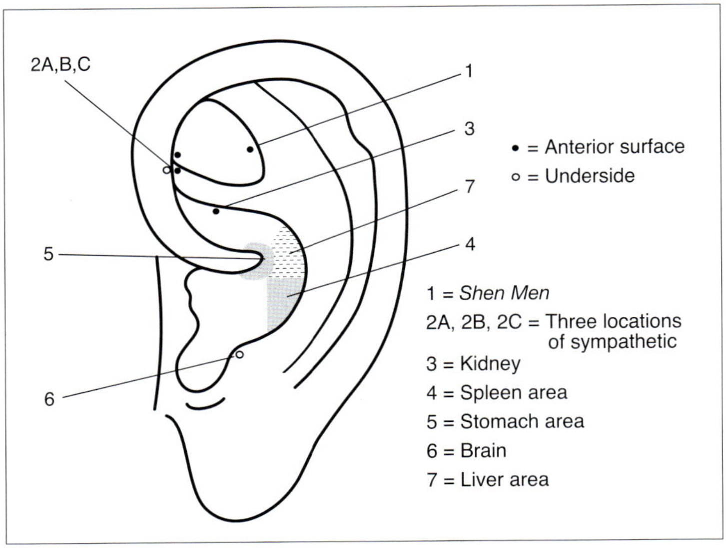

Fig. 7.**3** Ear acupuncture points for the elderly.

External Liniments

The application of external Chinese liniments to the skin of elderly patients is highly recommended as a treatment modality. The liniments are efficacious, pleasantly aromatic, and soothing because of their direct application to the body. Excellent liniments for elderly conditions and their specific use are outlined below:

- Woodlock Oil—an energetically warm oil that relaxes the sinews and muscles. It is effective for muscular aches and pains and is considered a primary oil for arthritis. Patients love Woodlock Oil.
- *Tieh Ta Yao Gin*—dispels blood and fluid stagnation, invigorates *qi* and blood, relaxes the tendons and muscles, promotes healing, and stops pain. Useful for traumatic injury, sprains, ligament tears, and bruises.
- *Po Sum On* Medicated Oil—relieves blood stagnation. Use for aches and pains due to wind-cold such as in the case of rheumatic joint pain. Apply often. Cover with gauze to prevent staining clothes.
- *Zheng Gu Shui*—its energetics are almost identical to *Tieh Ta Yao Gin* but additionally, as an energetically hot liniment, it penetrates to the bone level to promote bone regeneration and healing. Apply liberally but do not cover with a bandage or any other adhesive, as it will cause a burn to the skin. Overuse of *Zheng Gu Shui* can be drying.
- Regal Oil (*Kwan Loong*)—a cooling, aromatic, relaxing oil for painful conditions such as arthritis and other joint pain.

Consider where you apply the liniments. Keep them away from mucus membranes or hands that might touch mucus membranes. See Chapter 18 for a more detailed discussion of liniments.

Internal Herbs

Herbs available in patent, tincture, granular, or loose form can be effective choices for the elderly patient, however, you may not be able to use them without a physician's approval due to possible drug/herbal interactions. As always, check the suitability of the contents of the formula for the patient's condition. Dosages may need to be adjusted due to individual sensitivities. Be aware of possible side-effects such as allergic reactions, gas, bloating, itchy skin, etc. Check contraindications for patients with weak cardiovascular function.

Some herbs may promote loose stools and excess urination, which may cause "accidents." Assimilation of the herbs may be impaired due to weak central burner function of the aged. In short, while potentially therapeutic, the use of internal herbs may not be the most practical modality in a nursing home setting unless the aforementioned conditions can be avoided. If consent is given in writing, patent medicines are probably the most practical for their situation. Still, someone such as nursing home personnel will need to administer these at the appropriate frequency and dosage and monitor for side-effects.

Apart from the logistical problems of herbal dispensary, here are some other considerations when employing herbs. If you choose to administer herbs, beware of the possibility of causing negative herbal or drug/herbal interactions, the results of which are widely unknown. The best rule of thumb is not to combine herbal formulae and Western drugs at the same time, but to separate taking them by about 1 to 2 hours. Also, follow any other directions given by their licensed healthcare provider. When in doubt about herbal/drug interactions, do not administer the herbs.

However, judicious, skilled prescription can have enormous benefit for the patient. For the latest information on the largely unexplored area of herbal/pharmaceutical drug interaction, see John Chen's ground-breaking work. In one of his articles[3], John Chen lists many common Western medications and their pharmacological actions, and how these should be administered with Chinese herbs. It contains critical information all Oriental physicians using herbs should be aware of. Chen points out that according to the *Journal of the American Medical Association* (*JAMA*), it is estimated that 15 million adults in the United States in 1997 (18.4 % of all prescription users) took prescription drugs concurrently with herbal remedies and/or vitamins. Although herbal remedies are classified as dietary supplements, many of them possess strong medicinal properties and may affect the patients adversely if used incorrectly.

These possible interactions may affect the bioavailability or the clinical effectiveness of the substance, as well as the synergistic or antagonistic interactions between the herb/drug molecules. The highest risk of clinically significant interactions occurs between herbs and drugs that have sympathomimic effects, cardiovascular effects, diuretic effects, anti-coagulant, and anti-diabetic effects. Common herbs that have these pharmacodynamic interactions include *Herba Ephedrae* (*ma huang*)—sympathomimic; *Poria Cocos* (*fu ling*)—anti-diuretic; *Angelica Sinensis* (*tang gui*)—anti-coagulant; and *Atractylodes* (*gang zhu*)—anti-diabetic.

Herbal medications offer a host of benefits due to their biologic nature, which are useful in physically augmenting kidney vacuity, the overall historical diagnosis of aging. For an excellent resource to specifically treat many of the illnesses of aging with herbs see perhaps the two best works in this field—Lin and Flaws' work, *The Dao of Increasing Longevity*[7], in which Chinese herbal patent medicines are provided for hundreds of diseases and Yan De-Xin's *Aging and Blood Stasis*.[1]

Moxibustion

Moxibustion is a method of applying the Chinese herb *Artemisia Vulgaris* to the body to supplement, regulate, and invigorate the flow of *qi* and blood. While moxibustion in many cases is unrivaled in treating numerous conditions, it may not be permitted in institutional settings due to the smoke it creates, which could aggravate the respiratory function of other patients. Even the use of smokeless moxa may be precluded due to the presence of flammable oxygen in the facility. See Chapter 19 for a comprehensive discussion of moxibustion.

Massage

Massage is the procedure in which the body is stroked or rubbed in order to decrease tension and improves circulation. It is pleasant, therapeutic, and comforting on many levels. It is a good choice for these patients, however, the massage may need to be more focused on discrete body parts than administered in a full body session. Because muscular tone is usually poor, do not apply deep pressure. Take care not to bruise weakened patients.

Avoid massage in patients with deep vein thrombosis, which is a clotting problem of the veins of the lower extremities. Massage can potentially dislodge any clot and cause it to travel in particular to the lungs, resulting in a potentially life-threatening condition. Because this problem is often clinically silent and can only be diagnosed with sophisticated instrumentation such as duplex ultrasonography, venography, and CT venography, be aware of its common clinical manifestations, which include the following:

- a constant dull ache in the lower extremity;
- unilateral swelling of the ankle or calf;
- a sensation of warmth in the lower extremity;
- superficial venous dilation of the foot and anterior tibia;
- bluish discoloration of the foot or lower third of the leg;
- palpable thrombi;
- fever and/or tachycardia.

The elderly population is particularly suspect to this condition. Groups at high risk for massage to the legs include the following:

- those who have suffered pelvic fractures, acute head or spinal injury, stroke, total hip replacement surgery, or fractures of the lower extremities;
- those between the ages of 50 to 65;
- patients with atrial fibrillation, congestive heart failure, or myocardial infarction;
- burn patients or patients recovering from major orthopedic surgery;
- patients who are obese;
- patients with cancer of the lung, pancreas, or stomach;
- patients with certain blood and metabolic diseases.

Gwa Sha, Cups, Plum Blossom Needling, Bleeding

In general, avoid these modalities that are designed to vigorously activate the flow of *qi* and blood, or in the case of bleeding, to cool the blood as well. Elderly patients may be too weak for these modalities. If used at all, reserve these methods for those with strong constitutions. Table 7.**5** summarizes the use, contraindications and limitations of the treatment modalities discussed above.

The more we work with the elderly, the more likely we will understand their unique needs and adjust our treatment modalities accordingly. I have found that if we proceed cautiously, chances are we will promote more good than harm. Auricular medicine is certainly an area of practice that will turn into a specialization when practitioners work with these patients and assist in the codification of their results and experiences.

As with any patient, the conscientious practitioner's treatment plan must be circumscribed

Modalities	Generalized Therapeutic Use	Specific Clinical Conditions	Limitations, Contra-indications and Cautions
1. Infrared heat (with the TDP lamp or similar device)	Tonifies *yang* vacuity, increases metabolism and blood circulation	Night-time urination, insomnia, skin disorders, neurasthenia, arthritis, soft tissue injuries, sciatica, bedsores, musculoskeletal problems	Do not leave patient unattended during treatment due to the possible inability of the patient to report temperature sensation. Monitor heat by feeling affected area
2. Palpation	Confers the documented therapeutic benefits of touch	Lowers blood pressure, strengthens immunity, decreases pain, improves breathing, reduces anxiety and depression, increases emotional affect, lowers stress, relieves muscular tension	May not be perceived by patient as somewhat ineffective if vital *qi* is low
3. Scalp acupuncture	Musculoskeletal and nervous system disorders	Muscular atrophy, motor impairment, post-stroke sequelae, paralysis, involuntary movement disorders, multiple sclerosis	Requires patient to work with the practitioner to walk, move, etc. Patients are sometimes resistant to this or incapable of such movement

Table 7.**5** Treatment modalities: their therapeutic usage, limitations, and contraindications

Modalities	Generalized Therapeutic Use	Specific Clinical Conditions	Limitations, Contra-indications and Cautions
4. Electricity	*Bi*-(obstruction)syndromes	Arthritis, paralysis, pain	The "cold" nature of electricity is perhaps incompatible with *yang* vacuity syndromes. Sometimes jarring treatment for delicate, sensitive patients. Do not use on patients with heart conditions or pace-makers
5. Body needles	To regulate flow of *qi* and blood	Virtually any condition	Difficulty evoking *de qi* response. Difficulty with proper needle insertion due to patient condition, position i.e., wheelchair, bedridden, etc.
6. Auricular acupuncture	Adjusts the flow of *qi* and blood thereby reducing pain, moving stagnation, strengthening vital organs	Many illnesses: hypertension, vascular problems, chronic degenerative disorders, digestive disorders, osteoporosis, fatigue, poor balance, musculoskeletal problems, mental/emotional disorders	Avoid risk of infection by removing pellets; tacks (see Chapter 22) etc. in consideration of ear becoming wet from bathing, high humidity levels, etc. Monitor in patients with reduced wound-healing capacity
7. External liniments	Aromatic, relaxing/invigorating. See properties specific to each liniment	Muscular aches and pains, arthritis, joint pain, sprains, torn ligaments, bruises, rheumatic joint pain	Avoid eyes, mucous membranes, open wounds. For external use only
8. Internal herbs	For multiple benefits of herbs	For both internal and musculoskeletal diseases	Adjust dosage to individual sensitivity, condition etc. Consider possible herbal/pharmaceutical interactions and possible side-effects. Carefully monitor dosages
9. Moxibustion	Like acupuncture, to promote flow of *qi* and blood, strong *yang* tonic; for *zheng qi* vacuity, *correct* or *righteous qi* vacuity	Multiple illnesses especially those due to *yang* vacuity and cold	Aggravation of breathing or respiratory function. Do not use near oxygen tanks
10. Massage	Decreases tension, improves circulation	Full body or specific body parts	Caution not to bruise patient, patients may be delicate. Avoid with deep vein thrombosis (DVT) or patients at risk for it
11. *Gwa sha*, cupping, bleeding, plum blossom needling	Invigorates *qi* and blood, disperses blood stasis, drains heat/fire	Varicose veins, palpitations, tinnitus	Reserve for stronger patients. Avoid in patients with weakened constitutions

Table 7.**5** Treatment modalities: their therapeutic usage, limitations, and contraindications (cont.)

around the patient's condition. Due to their delicate condition and decreased vital *qi*, the elderly may not be eligible to receive many of the traditional modalities of Oriental medicine. However, comforting, compassionate care can be offered with Oriental medical therapies.

Hopefully, the fate of all of us is to grow old, but without the ravages of illness if we learn how to cultivate the vital *qi* and rebalance it. To age and die is a cohort of the *dao* (sometimes called *tao*, the natural path). To do so with grace, compassion, and strength can be one of our unique gifts to each other as human beings.

References

1. De-Xin Y. *Aging and Blood Stasis: A New TCM Approach to Geriatrics.* Boulder, CO: Blue Poppy Press; 1995:58.
2. Ibid.
3. Chen JK. Recognition and prevention of herb–drug interactions. *Amer J Acu.* 1999:6.
4. Cheung CS. Phlegm. *Ab Rev Clin Tra Chi Med.* June 1996:3.
5. Gardner-Abbate S. The differential diagnosis of pain in classical Chinese medicine: unique treatment approaches and acupoint energetics. *Amer J Acu.* 1996;24(4):269–284.
6. Acupuncture. *NIH Consensus Statement* 1999;15: 1–38.
7. Lin A, Flaws B. *The Dao of Increasing Longevity and Conserving One's Life.* Boulder, CO: Blue Poppy Press; 1991.

8 Help for Prolapsed Intervertebral Disks of the Lumbar Region (Herniated Disks)

Prolapse of intervertebral disks of the lumbar region, or lumbar herniation, is a frequent problem for which patients seek treatment. In Oriental medicine it has three etiologies:

1. injury to the local area;
2. invasion of wind, cold, or damp to an overtaxed condition; and
3. liver and kidney vacuity resulting in lack of nourishment to the channels.

Symptoms include radiative pain of the lower limbs, sensory disturbances to the same area, difficulty lifting the leg, and unilateral or bilateral sciatica. The pain may be severe or worse with lumbar flexion of the low back, and aggravated by a prolonged sitting or standing position in the dermatome area of the affected nerve root.

Normally, the intervertebral disk lies between the vertebral bodies of the spine and forms a mobile joint called a symphysis, which consists of the nucleus pulposus and an annulus fibrosus. The nucleus is a ball of transparent jelly, collagenous fibers, cells and mucopolysaccharides. The annulus fibrosus is made up of rings of fibers oriented in different directions, which surrounds the nucleus with a tough casting. The disks serve as shock absorbers of the forces of compression. The ability of the nucleus to become distorted, and the annulus fibrosus to bend, gives the vertebral bodies the ability to move on each other and to distribute the forces of compression. As we age, the nucleus tends to shrink, to become dry, and therefore less elastic and more fibrous. The annulus fibrosus concomitantly thickens and becomes more prone to rupture.

Technically speaking, a prolapsed disk refers to the herniation of the nuclear material due to tears in the annulus fibrosus. Pain and inflammation develop from pressure of the nuclear material on the posterior longitudinal ligament and the dura mater. The nerve root that can be affected is the one below the vertebra. The vertebral levels most subject to herniation are L4, L5, and S1. If the nerve root becomes affected, pain may be experienced in the corresponding dermatomal area and weakness and reduced reflexes may develop in the muscles. For an appreciation of this problem Figures 8.**1** and 8.**2** depict a normal and herniated disk, respectively.

The treatment plan for such a condition involves the breakdown and absorption of the herniated nuclear material and repair to the torn fibers of the annulus fibrosus and the posterior longitudinal ligament. In Oriental medicine, an effective treatment strategy for prolapsed intervertebral disks is a prescription called the Eight Needle Technique (see Chapter 6). Eight Needle

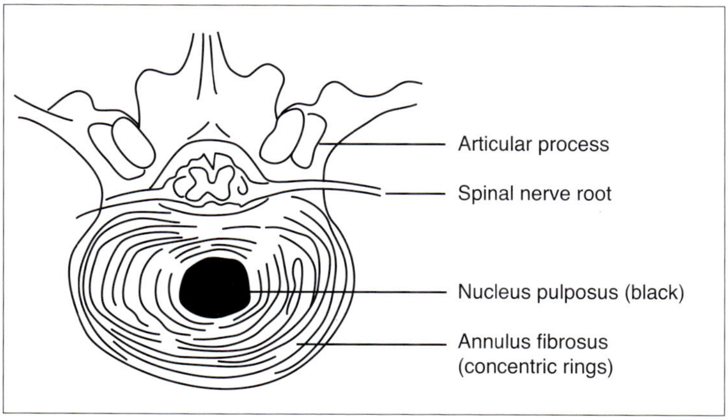

Fig. 8.**1** Normal intervertebral disk.

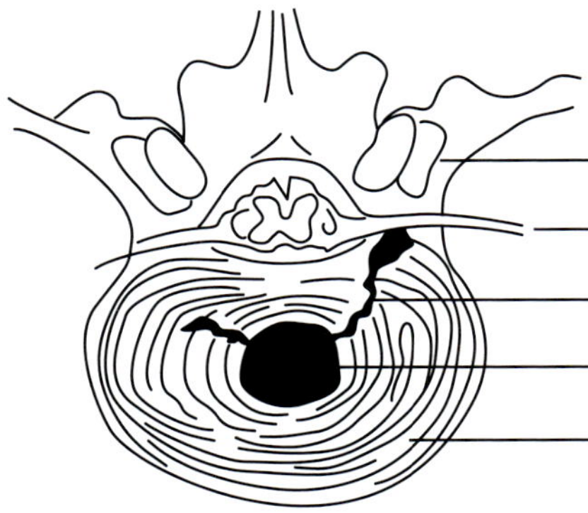

Fig. 8.**2** Herniated lumbar disk.

Points	Angles and Depths of Insertion (in)	Energetics
BL-23 (*shen shu*)	0.8–1.0 ppd. Moxa applicable	Back *shu* point of the kidney regulates the *qi* of the kidney (both kidney *yin* and *yang*). Resolves dampness in the lower burner. Strengthens the back. Nourishes kidney essence, benefits the bones and marrow. Nourishes blood
GV-4 (*ming men*)	0.5–1.0 ppd. Moxa applicable	Tonifies the original kidney *qi*, which is the person's condition, vitality, and genetic inheritance on a physical and mental level. Strengthens kidney *yang*. Strengthens the lower back, expels cold, dries damp-cold
BL-25 (*da chang shu*)	0.8–1.5 ppd. Moxa applicable	Back *shu* point of the large intestine eliminates stagnant *qi* and blood that may cause pain, numbness, muscular atrophy, and motor impairment of the back and lower extremities. Removes obstruction from the channel. Benefits the low back, back strain, pain in the sacroiliac joint and relieves fullness, swelling, and paralysis of the lower extremities
GV-3 (*yao yan guan*)	0.5–1.0 ppd. Moxa applicable	Tonifies kidney *yang* and *qi*. Strengthens the lower back and legs. Especially for backache that radiates to the legs. Pain in the lumbosacral region, numbness, muscular atrophy, motor impairment, weakness of the legs and knee pain caused by kidney *qi* and *yang* vacuity. Warms cold and dries damp
BL-40 (*wei zhong*)	0.5–1.5 ppd	*He* (uniting) point of the bladder channel. As the earth point, it is the controlling point of the channel. Clears dampness from the bladder channel. Eliminates blood stasis and channel obstruction that creates lower leg pain. Relaxes the sinews and tendons, opens the channel to benefit the lower back, knees, hips, and legs. For chronic or acute, excess or deficiency type backaches, but most effective for acute, excess backache that is either unilateral or bilateral, but not on the midline (on the spine)

Table 8.**1** The Eight Needle Point functions

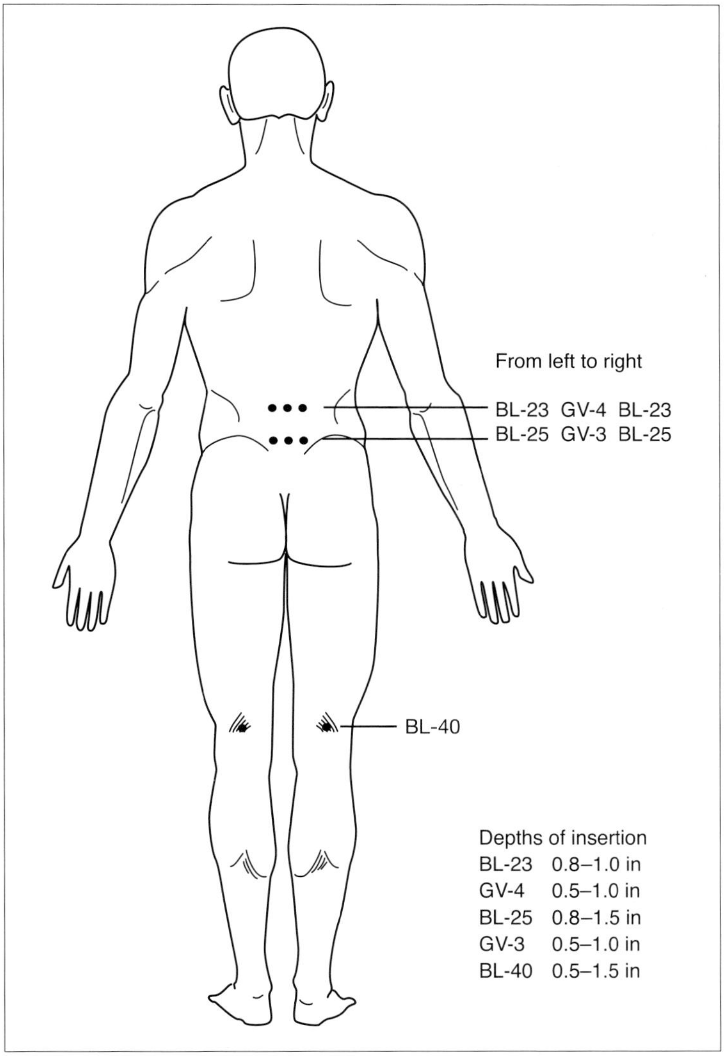

Fig. 8.**3** The eight needle points.

Technique is a Chinese treatment plan that is typically differentiated as clinically effective for kidney *qi* and *yang* vacuity resulting in low back pain. In its totality, it consists of eight points essentially in the local area of the herniation, or points with energetics primarily centered on remediating kidney *qi* and *yang xu* (*yang* vacuity). These points are BL-23 (*shen shu*) (bilateral), GV-4 (*ming men*), BL-25 (*da chang shu*) (bilateral), GV-3 (*yao yan guan*), and BL-40 (*wei zhong*) (bilateral). All of the points are located in the standard Chinese locations and needled to the standard Chinese depths of insertion. For clinical convenience, the points, angles, depths of insertion, and energetics are summarized in Table 8.**1** and depicted in Figure 8.**3**.

Position the patient as comfortably as possible on a treatment table by having them lie on their stomach. If this prone position makes their back uncomfortable, put a thick, firm pillow underneath their abdomen. This will take the pressure off their low back and open up the spine to assist in needle insertion.

While Bladder 23 and 25 may be needled in a perpendicular fashion, Chinese clinical experience has shown that an oblique insertion towards the spine is clinically effective to change the position of the prolapse and the neural roots, thereby reinforcing the therapeutic effect. All of the back points additionally have the function of easing pain, decreasing inflammation, activating blood flow, dredging the channels, and stimulating the nerve root directly. In this way the surrounding edema may be absorbed and the protrusion of the lumbar intervertebral disc rectified. The needle technique applied to each point depends upon whether the point needs to be tonified or dispersed. As in all cases of tonification and dispersion, needle retention times will vary, but as a general rule, retain the needles 20 minutes.

If the patient's back pain is correctly differentiated as due to prolapsed intervertebral disks of the lower extremities and Eight Needle Technique is applied, results are frequently efficacious and long-lasting with the added benefits accrued from tonifying kidney *qi* and *yang xu* of the body.

9 Thyroid Disorders, a Study in Contrasts

The Early Diagnosis and Treatment of Hypothyroidism

Hypothyroidism is a medical disorder that affects millions of people. It may be a functional disorder, the result of a weakened immune system, or produced iatrogenically by Western treatment such as a sequel to the treatment of hyperthyroidism. Factors that enter into weakening the immune system include nutritional deficiencies such as lack of iodine in the diet, deficiency of zinc, or deficiency of Vitamins E, A, C, B2, B6, selenium, or copper. Dietary excesses such as consumption of goitrogens (foods that block iodine utilization) such as excess peanuts, cabbage, soy, and mustard may be culprits, as well as lack of balanced, systemic exercise. While Western medicine has two differentiations of hypothyroidism—primary and secondary, the primary hypothyroidism is the most common.

Primary hypothyroidism is thought of as an autoimmune disease induced through chronic inflammation of the thyroid gland, also known as Hashimoto's thyroiditis. This variety occurs most commonly in women. Secondary hypothyroidism is caused by failure of the hypothalamus to regulate the thyroid gland, or lack of secretion of thyroid-stimulating hormone (TSH) from the pituitary gland. Laboratory evaluation is needed to differentiate these two varieties. Low levels of TSH exist in secondary hypothyroidism, whereas very high levels of TSH characterize primary hypothyroidism due to the fact that there is no feedback inhibition of the pituitary gland.

Signs and symptoms of the early diagnosis of primary hypothyroidism may be non-detectable except through blood analysis. Overt symptoms include fatigue, weight gain, problems of memory and concentration, lowered metabolism, hyperlipidemia, edema, cardiovascular changes, menstrual changes and hypertension.

Standard Western treatment generally involves lifelong hormonal replacement therapy with synthetic hormones or animal protomorphogens. In Oriental medicine, hypothyroidism is classified as a vacuity syndrome of *qi, yin* or *yang*, usually of the kidney, and this must be differentiated. Treatment can include long-term acupuncture and herbal medicine, nutritional supplementation, exercise, and avoidance of chemical exposure. Because the illness and not the person is treated in Western medicine the rest of the body may be affected to the point of even inducing hyperthyroidism as the dosage of the medication is experimented with. Oriental medicine treats the whole person such that overall the person remains healthier. In Western medicine the treatment is for life; in Oriental medicine it is based upon the presentation of signs and symptoms.

In my clinical experience I have treated many patients with hypothyroidism but rarely as a major complaint. Such patients came for other health problems and accepted their diagnosis of hypothyroidism and medication as a reality. They did not want it treated directly nor did they have any interest in its possible remediation.

One of my first opportunities to treat hypothyroidism was with a patient with an early diagnosis of primary hypothyroidism within 3 weeks of detection. The reason for this propitious early treatment was related to the vigilance of the patient whom I had been treating for the last 8 years, initially for the effects of stress on her health, and later for health maintenance and other minor problems. She always sought Oriental medical treatment for the resolution of her health problems and this case was no exception.

Following her annual exam with her physician, she came to see me about her new diagnosis of hypothyroidism. At the time of her visit to the doctor she reported to him that she felt she had been suffering from "flu" for about 3 months. The "flu" was characterized by fatigue, sore throat, cough and congestion. Her doctor, on what he called a hunch, ordered blood work that revealed that her thyroid-stimulating hormone level was 9.02, an amount that is almost twice the normal range of 0.40 to 5.50. He diagnosed her condition as primary hypothyroidism and wrote a prescription for Levoxyl and made recommendations for future appointments and periodic testing. However, he was very cooperative and supportive of her medical choices and encouraged her to receive Oriental medical treatment since he knew it to be her preferred approach.

When she came to see me 3 weeks later she did not have any overt, classical signs or symptoms of hypothyroidism. Subjectively she was experiencing tenderness in her neck. I conducted what I call a thyroid evaluation by gently palpating the following points bilaterally for tenderness: local points in the proximity of the thyroid gland, ST-9 (*ren ying*) and LI-18 (neck *fu tu*), and KI-3 (*tai xi*), the source point of the kidney, indicating kidney vacuity. All points were tender. In my experience such tenderness suggests a sub-clinical or clinical hypothyroid condition. I administered a treatment, whose protocol is found in Table 9.**1**. Its effect is to regulate and tonify the *qi* and *yang*, vitalize the blood, and stimulate and strengthen the immune system.

About a week later she returned for a treatment and said that her neck "felt good" and the treatment was repeated. Two weeks later she returned for her third treatment. Overall she felt better and described the previous treatment as a "jump start," an analogy I think accurately described the treatment plan and its desired effects.

One month after her initial acupuncture treatment her TSH levels were retested. They had almost halved from 9.02 to 4.98 and were now in the normal range of 0.40 to 5.50. Her doctor wrote on the lab results, "Great news!" For further reinforcement she received three acupuncture treatments over the next 3 months and then had a follow-up retest, which revealed that the TSH levels were now a little lower, 4.83. Her doctor pronounced the thyroid as normal and said "Great." My recommendation was to have her see me three to four times a year for health maintenance and continued monitoring of the thyroid gland.

As of the patient's 1-year evaluation, she has continued to maintain normal thyroid hormone levels and is in excellent health. I believe that the key to the successful resolution of this disorder is early detection, diagnosis, and treatment of the problem, augmented with high patient compliance, and of course the profound power of the medicine.

For clinician convenience, my treatment protocol follows in Table 9.**1**. It includes the points used, their locations and point energetics, as well as the specific needle technique employed. Insert needles in the order presented above. Retain the needles approximately 15 minutes. All needles are tonified after the *de qi* sensation is obtained. Use small amplitude of rotation as a tonification technique with #1 (36 g), 1 in (30 mm) Seirin needles. Remove needles in the same order as they were inserted.

Another patient then sought me out who had a similar diagnosis. She was a 61-year-old female who was diagnosed with hypothyroidism a month before consulting me. Her TSH level had recently risen from 4.5 to 6.37. Apart from high cholesterol, for which she was taking medication that worked, relatively speaking, she was very healthy. Her overall Oriental medical presentation pointed spleen and kidney *qi* and *yang* vacuity with concomitant liver *qi* stagnation due to blood vacuity as evidenced through long-standing cold hands and feet, sensitivity to external cold, gas, overthinking, minor seasonal allergies and a feeling of incompleteness with the bowel movement. Her tongue was slightly pale with paler sides and cracks. Her pulse was superficial, wiry, and weak in the lung and heart positions.

A physical examination by way of palpation revealed bilateral tenderness at ST-9 (*ren ying*), diagnostic of thyroid conditions, and Japanese "KI-3" (*tai xi*), referred to in Japanese acupuncture as the thyroid confirmation and treatment point. As the *yuan* source point KI-3 balances the kidney *yin* and *yang*, comprising the kidney *qi*, which was vacant. Her abdomen in the *dan tian* area was puffy and vacant indicating kidney *yang* vacuity. Palpation for a deep pulse at CV-6 (*qi hai*), where the *qi* of the two kidneys communicates with each other, was imperceptible, further supporting the vacuity of kidney *yang*. This could be construed, amongst other things in Western parlance, as hypothyroidism. (If interested in these concepts, see my book *The Art of Palpatory Diagnosis*[1] for more information on abdominal diagnosis and Japanese point location, energetics, and treatment.)

The first treatment was administered consisting of needling *yin tang*, the pituitary gland reflex point, to adjust the secretion of thyroid-stimulating hormone, ST-25 (*tian tu*) bilaterally to balance the *qi* and the blood, and KI-3 (*tai xi*) to tonify the kidney *qi*. All insertions were performed with a #1 gauge, 1 in Seirin needle. *Yin tang* was inserted

Points Used	Location	Energetics	Needle Technique
GV-20 (*bai hui*)	Standard Chinese location—7 *cun* within the anterior hairline, on the midpoint of the line connecting the apexes of the two auricles	Central reunion point—elevates the *yang*. Benefits the marrow (brain function, i.e., hormonal function)	Puncture 0.3–0.5 in horizontally in the direction of the channel, i.e., towards the face. Tonify
Yin tang	Standard Chinese location—midway between the medial ends of the two eyebrows	Reflex point of the pituitary gland that controls the thyroid gland	Puncture subcutaneously downward towards the nose 0.3–0.5 in. Tonify
Naganos	Find the ulna bone. Slide over it radially as you move towards Chinese LI-10 and LI-11. They are a group of four points located between the ulna bone and the large intestine channel. They are located about one fingerbreadth apart as you move distally from the elbow crease. Palpate each point deeply one at a time on each arm looking for the tenderest point on each arm. These are the points to be needled. (See Fig. 12.**2** in Chapter 12)	This group of four points is the Japanese equivalent to LI-11 (*qu chi*) and LI-10 (*shou san li*) and has similar energetics. They are powerful *qi* and blood tonics	Slowly insert perpendicularly to a depth of 0.5–1.0 in. Do not look for *qi*—search for a gummy, sticky feeling with the lift/thrust action of the needle. Do not tonify or disperse. Mechanically lift and thrust through the sticky area. Repeat two to three times. These points have a strong bearing down sensation on the arms and may be achy during and after treatment
Navel	Locate eight points equidistantly around the navel like points on a compass at a distance of 0.5 *cun* from the center of the navel	According to the *Nan Jing* text the navel pertains to the spleen; hence it can treat spleen problems. Because spleen is the figurative mother of lungs, it can treat lung pathology. As the figurative grandmother of kidney it can treat the kidney. Thus the cumulative effect of the points is to treat the three major organs pertaining to *qi*, the spleen, lung, and kidney	Puncture obliquely towards the navel 0.5 in. Tonify
SP-6 (*san yin jiao*)	Standard Chinese location—3 *cun* above the tip of the medial malleolus on the posterior border of the tibia on the line connecting the medial malleolus to SP-9 (*yin ling quan*)	Group *luo* of the three-leg *yin*—improves circulation, vitalizes the blood and tonifies liver, spleen, and kidney	Puncture perpendicularly 0.5–1.0 in bilaterally. Tonify
KI-7 (*fu liu*)	Standard Chinese location—2 *cun* directly above KI-3 (*tai xi*)	The metal point, therefore the tonification point of the kidney. Regulates the *qi* of the kidney, especially of the *yang*	Puncture perpendicularly 0.3–0.5 in bilaterally. Tonify

Table 9.**1** Hypothyroidism protocol

0.5 *cun* transversely downward, *tian tu* perpendicularly 0.8 in, and Japanese "KI-3" (which is identical to Chinese KI-5) transversely and posteriorly toward the heel 0.3 in. With the exception of KI-3, which was simply tonified by inserting the needle towards the heel, in the direction of the channel, which is a tonification technique, the other points were tonified with a slight clockwise turn of the needle, and needles were retained for about 15 minutes.

A prescription of Ginseng and *Astragalus* (also known as *Bu Zhong Yi Qi Tang* or Support the Central Qi) by Golden Flower Herbs was prescribed for a period of a month with a dosage of two pills, twice daily—one dose in the morning and one in the afternoon. The general purpose of the formula was to tonify the *qi* of the spleen and the kidney and to raise the *yang*.

After a month, the patient reported a feeling of well-being and decreased gas. Her blood work revealed a decrease in her TSH levels from 6.37 to 5.1, now within the normal range. Her doctor recommended a 6-month blood work follow up and I concurred. I likewise advised the patient to receive a minimum of one acupuncture treatment per month to maintain and/or further decrease the TSH level. During those times, further herbal evaluation and prescribing could be made based upon presenting signs and symptoms. Yearly Western thyroid evaluation was recommended to monitor TSH levels change in the blood so they can quickly be corrected.

Since then I have treated more hypothyroid patients similarly and with good result. For those I have treated with a longstanding diagnosis of hypothyroidism for 10–20 years, TSH levels have been reduced by about 67 % but at that point have been resistant to further lowering with Oriental medicine.

In summary, I am encouraged by the responsiveness of this disorder to Oriental medical intervention. As in the first case, I surmise that its efficacy is primarily related to early detection and appropriate differentiation and treatment and urge patients who receive such a diagnosis to seek qualified Oriental medical care and comply with practitioner recommendations to prevent a lifelong dependence on Synthroid or other thyroid medications and the possible devastating sequelae of hypothyroidism.

■ Hyperthyroidism

In contrast to hypothyroidism, which is relatively easier to treat with Oriental medical modalities, hyperthyroidism is almost as equally difficult to address. The difference of course stems from their etiology and the corresponding difference in correcting those causative factors.

As we recall from our understanding of *zang fu* pathology outlined above, hypothyroidism is caused by spleen or kidney *qi* and/or *yang* vacuity, liver *qi* stagnation and blood vacuity with its corresponding symptoms of lethargy, intolerance to cold, modest weight gain, forgetfulness and coarse dry skin. As we have seen, many times its symptoms are sub-clinical. The appropriate treatment plan is to tonify the *qi* and *yang* of the kidney, move the liver *qi* stagnation and tonify the blood.

Hyperthyroidism, with its symptoms of nervousness, increased sweating, hypersensitivity to heat, palpitations, fatigue, tachycardia, fidgeting, weight loss, insomnia, increased appetite and various eye symptoms such as photophobia, irritation and dryness is caused by a vacuity of the *yin* of the kidney and the liver and hyperactivity of liver *yang*. There may be heart *yin* vacuity symptoms as well. Energetically, on a continuum of *qi*, blood, *yin* and *yang*, *yin* is the deepest structural level and *qi* the most superficial, and hence we can see the reasons why hypothyroidism is more responsive to treatment than hyperthyroidism.

The doctors I studied with in China advocate the use of Western medications to treat hyperthyroidism although they do use some acupuncture as well. In my experience, because of the physical and psychological differences in both types of patients, i. e., the quiet and sedate hypothyroid patient versus agitated and restless hyperthyroid patient, the hyperthyroid patients are more resistant to therapy. In terms of acupuncture treatment, the hypothyroid patients who are vacuous in *qi* and *yang* can be well treated with needles and adjunct techniques such as moxibustion, the TDP lamp and herbs. Their symptoms of vacuity respond to energetic treatment better than symptoms of heat and fire, characteristic of hyperthyroidism.

For the hyperthyroid patient, reclining on the table in and of itself may be difficult because of the aforementioned symptoms. Because their deep-seated vacuity, their energy rises to the surface, so superficial needling should be avoided as well as long needle retention times. They are vacuous in a way more so than hypothyroid patients, because the *yin* is a deeper structural level. As such, hyperthyroidism takes longer to treat over time.

Below, two treatment plans are presented for the treatment of hyperthyroidism, which are similar in construction to each other, and can be used independently depending upon which modality you as a practitioner prefer or which therapy the patient would best tolerate.

Auricular Acupuncture

1. *Shen men*. This point, analogous to HT-7 (*shen men*) in the body, quiets the heart, grounds the patient, makes the heart serene, and puts the patient into a state of receptivity for treatment. It is useful for the heart *yin* vacuity symptoms of insomnia, restlessness, and agitation, tachycardia and palpitations. To accomplish this aim, treat this point first.
2. Kidney. Use to tonify kidney *yin* and liver *yin* because the kidney is the mother of liver. It will reduce fatigue and decrease fire by strengthening *yin*.
3. Liver. Use to directly nourish the liver *yin*, and to reduce the liver *yang* and fire, and move liver *qi* stagnation. The liver point treats eye symptoms, decreases nervousness, fidgeting and heat hypersensitivity.
4. Brain. Use to influence all neurological functions, to regulate the mind, and improve eye problems.

5–6. Spleen and stomach. Choose these points to tonify the *qi*, which produces the *yin* and the blood. The kidney *yin* will thereby be nourished through the five-element control cycle. Because these points relate to the earth element, they also ground and anchor the energy and this assists in treating insomnia, mental symptoms and appetite.

Method

After cleaning the ear with an alcohol swab, allow the ear to dry naturally. Then insert a 0.5 in #28 gauge needle perpendicularly into each point with the exception of the brain point, which is needled obliquely and anteriorly due to its location on the posterior border of the antitragus. Obtain *qi*, ideally in the form of heat, and tonify with a slight clockwise turn. Retain the needles 10 to 15 minutes. After removal of the needles, to reinforce the treatment, affix gold Magrain pellets to the same points but in the opposite ear, which has also been cleaned. Instruct the patient to press gently on the pellets three to five seconds, three to five times a day, for three to five days. Show the patient how to remove the pellets within the allotted timeframe or earlier if the ear becomes irritated, or to return to the office for you to remove them. See Figure 9.1 for the location of these points.

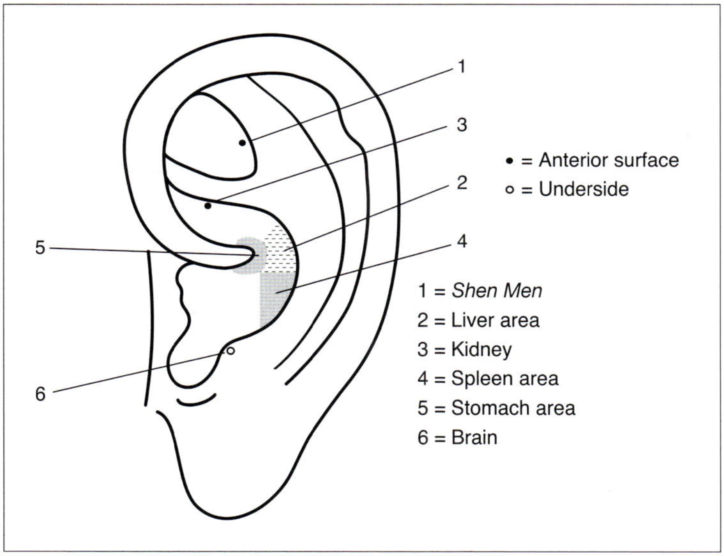

Fig. 9.**1** Auricular points to treat hyperthyroidism.

Body Acupuncture

Standard Chinese point locations are used for all points:

1. HT-7 (*shen men*). As the sedation point of the heart channel, this point quiets and stabilizes heart energetics manifesting as palpitations, tachycardia, restlessness, and insomnia. Puncture the point bilaterally and perpendicularly 0.3 to 0.5 in and tonify with a small clockwise twist. It is analogous to ear *shen men*.
2. ST-36 (*zu san li*). As the *he* (uniting) point of the stomach channel, ST-36 tonifies stomach and kidney *yin*. It reduces stomach fire leading to increased appetite. It builds blood, reduces fatigue, and weight gain. Puncture the point bilaterally and perpendicularly 0.8 to 1.2 in and tonify.
3. SP-6 (*san yin jiao*). As the group *luo* of the three-leg *yin*, *san yin jiao* nourishes the *yin* of the spleen, liver, and kidney. It improves dry symptoms of the eyes, builds blood, and grounds the patient. Puncture SP-6 perpendicularly and bilaterally 0.5 in. Try to direct the *de qi* sensation to KI-1 (*yong quan*) by placing your thumb above SP-6 to block the *qi*. Then tonify the point.
4. LR-3 (*tai chong*). According to the Chinese, this is the best point to tonify the *yin* of the liver. Concomitantly, it reduces liver *yang* rising because source points have this function. It decreases nervousness and treats various eye disorders. Needle the points bilaterally, obliquely, and proximally (i. e., away from the toes), 0.3 to 0.5 in in the direction of the channel and stimulate mildly.
5. KI-3 (*tai xi*). The Chinese claim Kidney 3 is better than Spleen 6 to support the *yin* of the body, thereby reducing fatigue and reducing fire. Puncture Kidney 3 perpendicularly 0.3 in.
6. GB-1 (*tong zi liao*). For symptoms of eye involvement, pinch the skin to insert the needle, then direct laterally and horizontally 0.2 to 0.3 in along the skin.
7. BL-2 (*zan zhu*). Bladder 2 is also effective for the various eye symptoms associated with hyperthyroidism. It soothes the liver, assists in nourishing the eyes and reinforces the kidney. Pinch the skin in the eyebrow area and puncture the point horizontally 0.3 in towards the lateral aspect of the face.

Exercise and herbs are also helpful support systems in the treatment of hyperthyroidism and emotional factors should be explored with the patient. As always it is also important to provide patient, caring treatment and to offer behavioral recommendations about lifestyle factors that consume essence and promote the development of the fire in the body.

Reference

1. Gardner-Abbate S. *The Art of Palpatory Diagnosis in Oriental Medicine*. London: Churchill Livingstone; 2001.

10 The Management of Multiple Sclerosis with the Extraordinary Vessels

As practitioners and fellow humans, we know that there is no secret to the suffering of patients with multiple sclerosis (MS). It is a devastating chronic illness, which robs the patient of control over simple physiological processes, often to the point of physical incapacitation. While its myriad signs and symptoms can be recognized once the illness has progressed, its origins are as mysterious as they are insidious.

From a Western perspective MS is characterized by demylinated nerve sheaths of the central nervous system, which consequently result in a lack of fluid nervous transmission, such that indications of nervous system failure result. These symptoms include lack of motor control, problems with walking and control of limbs, intestinal and bladder incontinence, and visual disturbances. Other disturbing developments include memory and concentration problems, extreme fatigue, and lack of sexual energy.

With regard to Western prognosis and treatment, multiple sclerosis is characterized by recurrent periods of exacerbation of symptoms. The disease may progress pathologically to the point of immobilization and confinement, although at times the patient may experience spontaneous and unexplained remissions. There is no treatment, there is no cure, and prognosis is poor. Experimentation with various diets, largely those that eliminate sugar and food allergens, raw foods diets, and those that reduce meat, carbohydrates, and saturated fat, yield varied and/or temporary results, as does stress reduction, mild exercise, and a positive mental attitude.

Up until about 30 years ago, MS was unheard of in China. It first became noticed in large, populated cites. The assumption was advanced that the illness was due to the stress of modern culture as well as the concomitant pollution of contemporary times. Chinese medical theory, inferring from signs and symptoms, advanced that overall, MS was a problem of *yin* vacuity that originally began with fire in the metal element at an early age. Fever such as scarlet fever, fever accompanying German measles, or other fevers of unexplained origin, were often considered the causative factor that then devolved into other organs' vacuity of *yin*, such as *yin* vacuity of the kidney and the liver.

Interestingly, heat seems to aggravate the condition, a further substantiation that the *yin* of the body is truly involved. Pathology progresses according to the reverse *sheng* cycle (opposite to the normal nourishing cycle of the five elements) thus revealing the element and organ disharmonies that will ensue. As water disharmonies develop, the patient is near the end of the elemental cycle where it finally terminates in a return to metal and the extinction of *qi* or death.

While obviously nothing can be done for this scorching of the *yin* aspect of metal, still Oriental medicine posits a 40% chance of success with treatment, which is better than a zero prognosis by Western doctors. In some cases this edge can take the patient to the point of remission, and in others to that of management of the illness's symptoms, much akin to a pain management protocol, to the point that the patient can cope with many of the symptoms of MS. Treatment needs to be frequent, lifestyle factors adopted like sensible Chinese dietary therapies, and gentle exercise such as stretching, and stress reduction mechanisms implemented.

Oriental medical practitioners may select various places to begin treatment. Treating the manifestation or the branch usually has short-term success. Treating the root and the branch is an option that works better, but beware of too many needles (greater than ten), which can drain the patient's energy. In my experience with MS patients as well as with any patient, treating the root not only works faster but also produces results that are more sustainable.

Various modalities may be employed but my preferred methods are ear therapy with gold Magrain pellets on the major organs involved, such as lung, kidney, spleen, stomach, liver, and brain as a core formula and *shen men*.

Body acupuncture, with a protocol practitioners may be well aware of but not utilize, is that of the *jing* treatment. The Chinese *jing* treatment is a therapeutic strategy that makes use of the master and coupled points of the eight extraordinary vessels plus CV-6 (*qi hai*) to activate the functions of the extraordinary vessels. Remember that the extraordinary vessels are not subject to the same laws of *yin/yang* that characterize the 12 main channels. While they have numerous physiological functions, in essence they are homeostatic vessels, which first can supplement vacuity when needed, especially of *jing*, which is vacuous in MS patients, and second they can reduce excesses and pathological products such as phlegm, damp, stagnant *qi*, and blood that develop due to underlying vacuities.

Many clinicians are wary of using the extraordinary vessels for fear of draining an already weakened patient, but a clear understanding of the physiology of the extraordinary vessels and centuries of clinical experience as well as your own proves this fear is unfounded. Consult Table 10.**1** for a summary of the generalized functions of each of the extraordinary vessels.

The *jing* treatment contacts the *qi* of the patient on a very deep level, that of the *jing qi*, which is a combination of one's pre- and post-natal *qi*—in short, who we are. By virtue of the needles the *jing* treatment accesses this very deep core energetic substrate and augments it, frees it up and circulates it for proper physiological functioning. Patients with multiple sclerosis describe the effect of this treatment as like a rested vacation—certainly a testimony to the power of the needles and the energetic zones regulated by the extraordinary vessels.

Treatment may be administered daily or from two to five days per week depending upon the pa-

Functions		Usages
1. Homeostatic	Absorbs excess perverse energy from the 12 main channels	To treat fever caused by invasion of an external pathogen
2. Circulatory	Warms and defends the surface by circulating *wei qi*	To increase *yang* in body
3. Enriching	Enriches the body with *qi*, blood, and ancestral *qi*	To treat vacuities in those areas
4. Controlling	Serves as reservoirs and conductors of *jing*	To treat essence vacuity illness and the developmental lifecycle problems
5. Nourishing	Harmonizes and nourishes the extraordinary organs of the gall bladder, uterus, brain, blood vessels, bone marrow, and bone	To treat diseases of the liver/gall bladder, uterus, brain, blood vessels, bone marrow, and bone
6. Supervisory	Exerts a commanding role over areas of the body, essential substances, and *zang fu* organs	To treat zones of the body, essential substances, and *zang fu* organs
7. Balancing	Regulates energy	a. When the pulses are balanced but the patient still complains of symptoms b. When the 12 main channels have failed c. To treat the root causes of a disease
8. Supplementing	Supplements multiple vacuities	To treat chronic disease, metabolic and hormonal disorders, and psychic strain
9. Adjusting	Reduces inherited or acquired structural stress	To treat muscle tension, postural, or structural stress

Table 10.**1** The general function of the extraordinary vessels

tient's condition, availability, or other factors. Needles are inserted in the order from top to bottom to ground and anchor the *qi*, and from right to left to bring the *yin* into the *yang*, and unilaterally. See Table 10.**2** for which side of the body to treat, as well as my adjusted angles and depths of insertion. Standard Chinese point locations are employed.

Use #1 gauge 30 mm Seirin needles for patient comfort and in consideration of their vacuous condition. Simply insert each needle, obtain no-to-little *qi*, and twist once in a small clockwise direction for tonification. Retain the needles for 10 to 15 minutes.

Before you leave the room, instruct the patient to try not to think of anything, but if they must, to think about the needles tapping into the deepest reserves of the body for replenishment and healing. After the treatment the patient should report a feeling of deep-seated energy, calmness, and lack of pain. Instruct the patient to go home and rest instead of expending any energy acquired by the treatment.

The patient should not feel light-headed, spacey, weak, shaky, or very tired. If any of these scenarios develop, check your needle size, insertion technique, angle and depth of needle insertion, needle manipulation and retention time, any of which may be faulty. Allow the patient to rest five to ten minutes in the treatment room after treatment, to get up slowly, and offer them a small glass of water or hot tea before they leave as their energy has been contacted at a very deep level.

This is an easy-to-use treatment protocol that treats the root of the disorder by supplementing and regulating the *qi*. It works on a profound level physically, energetically, and emotionally. Stick with it as an effective treatment strategy for the management of multiple sclerosis. As improvement is made, other points may be substituted

Point Order	Eight Curious Vessel Master Point	Eight Curious Vessel Coupled Point	Side of the Body to Needle	Needle Technique (Japanese needles best, #1 g)
TB-5 (*wai guan*)	*yang wei mai*	GB-41 (*zu lin qi*)	Right side	Perpendicular superficial insertion 0.3 in. No or small manipulation depending upon patient's condition
GB-41 (*zu lin qi*)	*dai mai*	TB-5 (*wai guan*)	Left side	Obliquely 0.3 in. In the direction of the channel (towards the toe)
PC-6 (*nei guan*)	*yin wei mai*	SP-4 (*gong sun*)	Left side	Superficial insertion 0.3 in. No or light manipulation depending upon patient's condition
SP-4 (*gong sun*)	*chong mai*	PC-6 (*nei guan*)	Right side	Perpendicular or oblique insertion 0.3 in. If oblique, needle in direction of channel
LU-7 (*lie que*)	*ren mai*	KI-6 (*zhao hai*)	Right side	Obliquely 0.3 in towards thumb
KI-6 (*zhao hai*)	*yin qiao mai*	LU-7 (*lie que*)	Left side	Posteriorly horizontally 0.1 – 0.2 in in direction of channel (towards the heel)
SI-3 (*hou xi*)	*du mai*	BL-62 (*shen mai*)	Left side	Perpendicular or obliquely upward (distally) 0.2 – 0.3 in
BL-62 (*shen mai*)	*yang qiao mai*	SI-3 (*hou xi*)	Right side	Obliquely 0.2 – 0.3 in in the direction of the channel (towards the toes)
CV-6 (*qi hai*)	X	X	Center	Perpendicularly 1.0 – 1.5 in. Summon the *qi* to the area and tonify

Table 10.**2** Eight confluent point protocol

based upon the energetic layer affected, and acute and transient symptoms, but always try to see where the symptoms are coming from for more long lasting results.

Acupuncture will not cure multiple sclerosis as it does not cure many other devastating illnesses. The weakness, pain, and debilitation of multiple sclerosis can co-exist amidst the joy and splendor of life and can be managed through the physical, mental, and emotional relief acupuncture can bring by the correct discernment and treatment of energetic layers involved. That relief can be a lifeline of hope to many patients and to you as a practitioner.

11 The Pathophysiology and Treatment of Peripheral Neuropathy of the Upper and Lower Extremities

Whether it be a sequel to AIDS, diabetes, cancer therapies, or alcoholism; hereditary, toxic, metabolic, infectious, inflammatory or ischemic diseases, peripheral neuropathy (or polyneuritis), is an insidious condition that causes much suffering to millions of people.

The peripheral nervous system consists of the nerves that connect the central nervous system to the muscles and internal organs, and transmit sensation throughout the body, thereby making feeling possible. The main clinical manifestations of peripheral neuropathy include pain, aching, burning, numbness, and tingling of the distal limbs, as well as itching or even extreme sensitivity to even the slightest touch. Frequently, these symptoms are bilateral, exacerbated at night, and affect the lower limbs more than the upper limbs. Typical Western treatment revolves around relieving patient discomfort.

All of the aforementioned diseases have in common a severe vacuity of *yin*, blood, and *qi* such that static blood is engendered. Since the etiology of most of this blood stagnation is *qi*, blood, or *yin* vacuity, for long-lasting results, these causative factors must likewise be addressed along with the treatment strategy to invigorate the blood. Regardless of whether one is using acupuncture or an herbal prescription the correct treatment entails addressing the etiological factors. From an acupuncture perspective there are certain unique therapies that can benefit this condition, particularly those treating blood stasis. Acupuncture points with known clinical efficacy can then be added to the core treatment to address underlying deficiencies.

Traditional acupuncture treatment approaches have concentrated on the use of local points, *luo* and *shu* (stream) points of the affected channels to treat peripheral neuropathy. In my treatment of peripheral neuropathy of the lower limbs I use five core points—KI-1 (*yong quan*), LR-4 (*zhong feng*), SP-6 (*san yin jiao*), GB-34 (*yang ling quan*), and KI-6 (*zhao hai*). For the upper extremities I rely on PC-6 (*nei guan*), LU-9 (*tai yuan*), LI-11 (*qu chi*), ST-12 (*que pen*) and CV-17 (*shan zhong*).

To determine their applicability in treatment, palpate each point, one at a time, for any noticeable tenderness that the patient may report to you. Press the point in a rubbing motion for about 3 seconds to the depth that you would actually needle. If the point is tender it can be needled in treatment. The energetics of these points as well as their corresponding needling techniques and locations, some of which are Japanese locations, are summarized in Table 11.**1** and illustrated in Figures 11.**1** and 11.**2**.

Point	Energetics	Needle Technique
Lower limb		
KI-1 (*yong quan*)	Promotes blood circulation. Invigorates *qi*; regulates flow of *qi*. Clears heat. Activates collaterals. Promotes production of body fluid	Puncture perpendicularly 0.3 – 0.5 in with a #1 gauge needle. Patients should be taught to press the point on a daily basis for several minutes. Continue daily until there is no more tenderness
LR-4 (*zhong feng*)	As the metal point on a wood meridian, it moves *qi* and blood, because metal controls wood via the five element control (*ko*) cycle. Primary point for blood stagnation in the lower burner analogous to PC-6 (*nei guan*) in the upper burner	Puncture perpendicularly 0.3 – 0.5 in or obliquely upward in the direction of the liver channel. Can be rubbed firmly by patient for self-treatment

* Overall treatment: to promote blood circulation and remove blood stasis; to supplement the *qi*, blood, and *yin*.

Table 11.**1** Primary treatment points for peripheral neuropathy of the lower and upper limbs*

Point	Energetics	Needle Technique
SP-6 (*san yin jiao*)	As group *luo* of the three-leg *yin* it nourishes the *yin* of the liver, spleen, and kidney. Improves circulation in the lower burner. For poor venous circulation	Puncture perpendicularly 0.5 – 1.0 in
KI-6 (*zhao hai*)	Nourishes the *yin*, cools the blood. Reduces inflammation. Supports the sympathetic nervous system	Puncture transversely 0.1 in towards the heel with a #1 gauge needle. Do not obtain *qi*
GB-34 (*yang ling quan*)	As the influential point that dominates the tendons, it is a primary point for tendons, muscles, ligaments, and nerves	Puncture perpendicularly 0.8 – 1.2 in. Have the patient rub with strong pressure
Upper limb		
PC-6 (*nei guan*)	Removes stagnation anywhere in the body. Can drain off excess stuck energy of upper burner. Produces *yin* and blood	Puncture perpendicularly 0.5 – 1.0 in or apply deep dispersive pressure by hand, especially on the left side
LI-11 (*qu chi*)	As a powerful blood tonic, builds blood, clears heat and fire. Benefits the sinews. Boosts *qi*	Puncture perpendicularly 0.5 – 1.0 in
ST-12 (*que pen*)	Loosens tissues and muscles of the supraclavicular fossa to promote *qi* and blood flow through this critical nexus over the brachial plexus, which supplies the blood and nerves of the upper extremities, neck and face	Puncture perpendicularly 0.3 – 0.5 in, avoid the transverse cervical artery. Needle with caution as this point is on the apex of the lung. Alternative technique is with patient lying on their side to puncture perpendicularly toward the spine
LU-9 (*tai yuan*)	As the *shu* (stream) and *yuan* (source) point—useful for distal extremities and chronic conditions. As the influential point that dominates the vessels (union of veins and arteries), improves circulation by benefiting arteries	Puncture perpendicularly 0.2 – 0.3 in
CV-17 (*tan zhong*)	Opens the chest, adjusts *qi*, spreads the *qi*. One of the eight influential points that dominates the *qi*	Puncture transversely upward (toward the head in the direction of the channel) 0.3 – 0.5 in. Retain needles 10 – 15 minutes
Contraindications/ instructions	**Do not use** any of these points in pregnancy due to their strong ability to move the blood, or with patients who have a history of deep vein thrombosis of the lower limbs	

Table 11.**1** Primary treatment points for peripheral neuropathy of the lower and upper limbs (cont.)

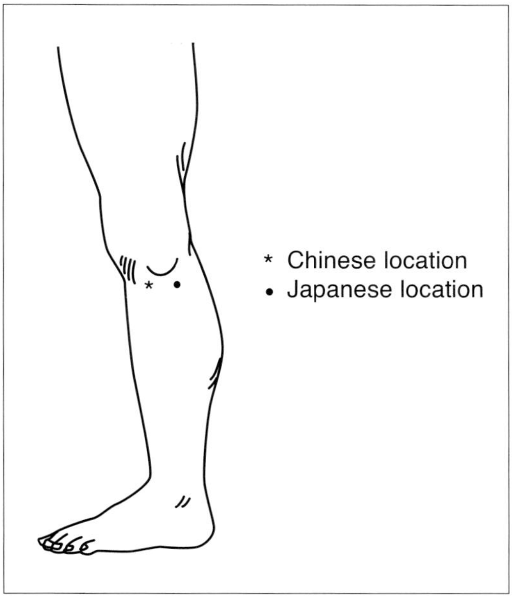

Fig. 11.**1** Two locations of GB-34 (*yang ling quan*).

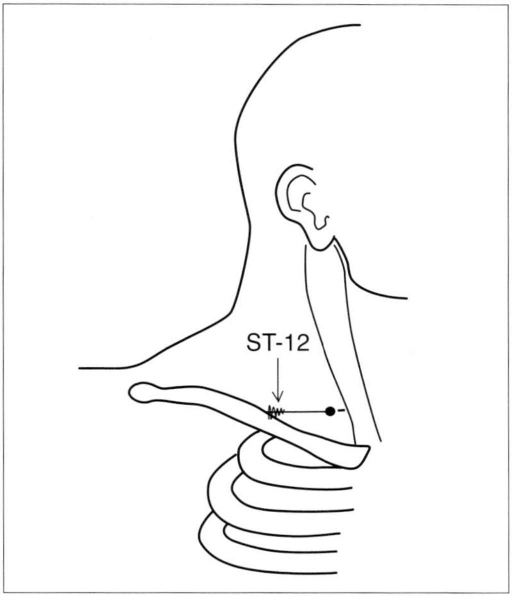

Fig. 11.**2** Location of ST-12 (*que pen*), regional anatomy, and needle placement.

As part of self-treatment, the patient can also apply the Chinese liniment *Zheng Gu Shui* to the affected areas. *Zheng Gu Shui* is the most powerful Chinese prepared liniment in that it has the strongest ability to penetrate the skin deeply, thus making it the liniment of choice for moving blood stagnation.

Apply *Zheng Gu Shui* generously before bedtime with a cotton ball and let it dry, as the liquid can stain clothes. Do not apply the liniment near open wounds, on irritated skin, ulcerated tissue, or near mucous membranes. Discontinue use if irritation or excessive dryness develops.

An additional effective treatment modality includes the use of the plum blossom needle to the areas where the neuropathy occurs. Lightly tap the skin surface starting distally and moving up the legs or arms in the direction of venous circulation and repeat. Do this for about 3 minutes. This hammering technique can be slightly discomforting to the patient but if tolerated it is an effective strategy. Some slight blood extravasation in the form of small droplets may occur as a result of the tapping; this is both normal and therapeutic. You can give or sell the patient a plastic disposable plum blossom needle with which to treat him/herself at home on a daily basis to speed up the effect. Instruct the patient on how to use and dispose of the tool properly and instruct them only to use it on themselves to prevent the transmission of infectious disease.

The use of these ten powerful points, augmented with an external liniment and ancillary techniques, constitute an effective treatment for the clinical manifestations of peripheral neuropathy and its underlying pathologies of blood stasis, *qi*, blood and *yin* vacuity, and can bring much relief.

12 Prolapses: A Beneficial Treatment with Oriental Medicine

The development of prolapses of various organs is a natural human condition. Prolapses develop from a weakened physical condition, age, gravity, excess weight, various childbirth situations, organ removal, or organ weakness. In Chinese medicine, prolapses are primarily viewed as being related to sinking spleen *qi*. In Japanese theory, this concept is expressed in slightly different ways, ultimately as being related to weak immunity (a component of which is spleen *qi*, our source of post-natal nourishment), as well as kidney *qi* vacuity. The essential Oriental medical treatment plan revolves around raising the *yang*, or the *qi* of the spleen.

Prolapses may occur in several parts of the body. Common sites involve the rectum, bladder, uterus, and intestines. Incompetent sphincters that allow for acid reflux disease, hiatal hernia, inguinal hernias, and even mitral valve prolapse of the heart fall within the domain of prolapses.

Patients may come to be treated for these conditions as their major complaint, or the prolapse may be a symptom that is part of their medical history. In any event, prolapses can be addressed with an Oriental treatment strategy if the prolapse is not at the point where it needs to be repaired surgically. The modalities most suited for this condition include needles, moxibustion, and the TDP lamp (therapeutic infrared lamp).

While each type of prolapse has specific points that are clinically effective for its specific differentiation, a core outline of points that one could use to treat prolapses, and then augment or modify based on signs and symptoms, includes KI-27 (*shu fu*), ST-13 (*qi hu*), GV-20 (*bai hui*), LR-5 (*li gou*), and a special group of points known as the *naganos*. Let us look at the unique energetics of this group of points and discuss their needling techniques.

Energetics

Kidney 27 (*shu fu*) is the last point on the kidney channel. Energetically, it is classified as the *shu* of *shu* points. Remember that according to Oriental medical theory, a *shu* point can monitor and treat aberrations of the *qi* and blood. Being the *shu* of *shu* points means it is very important, a master *shu* point so to speak. It has the energetic effect of adjusting the *qi* and blood of all the organs. KI-27 is located 2 *cun* lateral to the *ren* channel, on the lower border of the clavicle. To determine the need to needle this point, rub each point separately for about 3 seconds in a transverse manner. The point typically elicits an achy sensation, indicating that it could benefit from treatment.

Stomach 13 (*qi hu*) is located close to KI-27. It is found 4 *cun* lateral to the *ren* channel on the lower border of the clavicle. In Japanese acupuncture, ST-13 is considered the most important point in the treatment of prolapses, analogous to GV-20 in Chinese acupuncture. A loose translation of ST-13's name in Japanese is "cause a reversal," hence its applicability to the treatment of prolapse to reverse the collapsed condition. This translation is somewhat similar to the Chinese translated name, "*Qi's* Household," which designates that ST-13 is a site of intersection of the stomach, large intestine, triple warmer, small intestine, and many other divergent channels, hence its ability to raise the *yang*.

In Chinese acupuncture Governing Vessel 20 (*bai hui*) is perhaps the most well known point for the treatment of prolapse. Located 5 *cun* within the anterior hairline on the governing vessel channel, it has the ability to raise the *yang*, especially with the use of moxibustion.

Liver 5 (*li gou*) is an additional point that can be treated, especially if the prolapse is liver-related, as in the case of inguinal hernia or uterine prolapse. As the *luo* point of the liver channel, LR-5 can be used as a longitudinal *luo* to stimulate the organ and channel of the liver. The liver channel encircles the external genitalia, connects to the

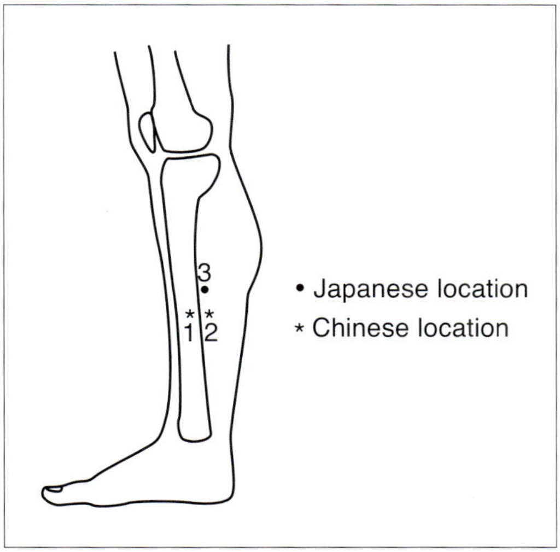

Fig. 12.**1** Three locations of LR-5 (*li gou*).

uterus, and dominates the tendons, muscles, ligaments, and nerves. Liver 5 has three potential locations, which are shown in Figure 12.**1** and are described below in the section on needling.

The *naganos* are a special group of points that can be needled in the treatment of prolapse. They are in close proximity to LI-11 (*qu chi*) and LI-10 (*shou san li*) and have equivalent energetics. In essence they are the Japanese locations of those points. As the *he* (uniting) point of the large intestine and upper *he* (uniting) point of the stomach respectively (meaning they are the sources of post-natal *qi* that strengthen organ *qi* and produce blood to nourish tendons and muscles), these points are powerful *qi* and blood tonics.

To locate the *naganos*, which run parallel to the areas of LI-10 and LI-11, find the ulna bone close to LI-11 and slide over it towards the medial side of the arm. The *naganos* are located between the ulna bone and the large intestine channel. These four points are located about one fingerbreadth apart as you move distally from the elbow crease. Palpate the *naganos* one point at a time, one side at a time, to find the tenderest point on each arm.

Needling

Prior to needling, palpate all of these points in a manner similar to that described under KI-27 as physical verification of their involvement with the prolapse. See Figures 12.**1** and 12.**2a,** and **b** for the locations of Liver 5 and *naganos* respectively.

Palpate the three locations of Liver 5 (LR-5, *li gou*) in the following way:

- (Location 1—Chinese): 5 *cun* above the medial malleolus vertically in the cleft on the medial border of the tibia. Palpate vertically in the cleft.
- (Location 2—Chinese): 5 *cun* above the medial malleolus on the posterior border of the tibia. Palpate vertically off the bone.
- (Location 3—Japanese): Midway between the tip of the medial malleolus and SP-9 (*yin ling quan*) on the posterior border of the tibia. Palpate vertically off the bone.

Both KI-27 and ST-13 are needled in the same manner, transversely toward the lateral aspect of the chest, 0.3 to 0.5 in. An efficient technique I have adopted is to connect the two points by way of threading, or "through-and-through" needling. This reduces the number of needles normally required from four to two. Insert the needle into KI-27 and thread toward ST-13 in a transverse subcutaneous manner. Use caution by not obtaining *qi*, and not using a lift-thrust method, due to the proximity of the lungs and the potential of causing a pneumothorax.

Bai hui has a number of needling techniques, depending on its use. In the treatment of prolapse, I needle the point obliquely at a 15 to 45 ° angle in the direction of the channel: that is, anteriorly, which is a tonification technique because this is the direction of the channel. Insert the needle 0.5 in in this manner. A small amount of *qi* may be obtained. If moxa, the method of choice, is used, burn three moxa cones on the point in a direct, non-scarring method, or warm with a moxa pole. Use caution not to burn the head hair.

Choose the tenderest LR-5 location. Each point is needled the following way: LR-5 locations 1 and 3—needle 0.3 to 0.5 in proximally in the direction of the channel; LR-5 location 2—needle transversely 0.3 to 0.5 in toward the inner leg. A small amount of *qi* may be obtained on the selected point.

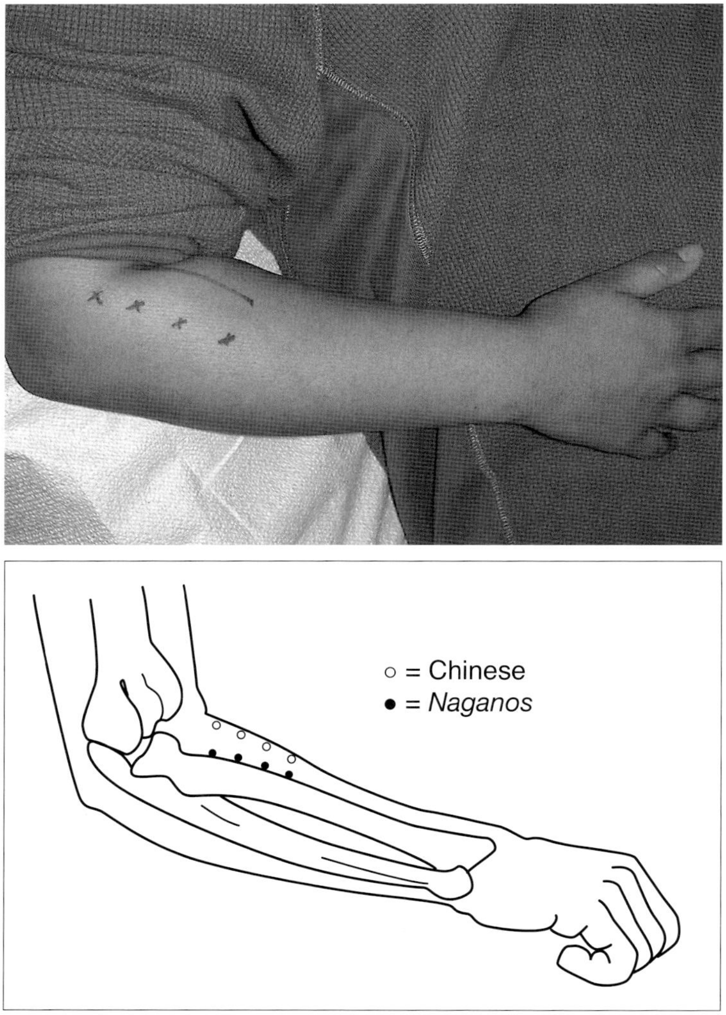

Fig. 12.**2a, b** The *naganos* (x) and their relationship to LI-10 (*shou san li*) and LI-11 (*qu chi*).

The tenderest *nagano* point on each arm can be needled. Insert the needle perpendicularly 0.5 to 1 in. Do not obtain *qi*; rather, lift and thrust gently but repeatedly to break through areas of calcification that develop in these points. Here you are using the needle to mechanically break up obstruction in the area, which tends to be "gummy" at first, then "crunchy" as you break up the gumminess. This technique produces a strong bearing-down sensation in the arm during needling, and achiness after treatment. Repeat the lift-thrust technique two to three times during treatment.

As mentioned previously, other points may be added to the core treatment plan. Likewise, indirect moxibustion can be applied to all of these points for 3 to 5 minutes. An extra modality I find effective for abdominal prolapses is to apply the TDP lamp over the abdomen for period of 20 minutes per session. This treatment is valuable for prolapses such as that of the bladder, uterus, and intestines. The effect of the lamp serves to strengthen kidney *qi*, whose natural energy rises and supports the *qi* of the spleen to hold things in place.

In my clinical experience, all of these modalities have proven successful in individual cases for complete remediation of the prolapse, or at least to help stabilize the condition if it has not progressed to the point of requiring surgical intervention.

13 The Treatment of Seasonal Affective Disorder (SAD): Classical Points for a Contemporary Condition

Seasonal Affective Disorder, a variety of depression, is a debilitating problem that interferes with the quality of life of thousands of people, especially during the fall, winter, and early spring months when there is less light than in the summer months. This syndrome seems to be a worldwide phenomenon occurring cross-culturally, especially in countries not close to the equator. Clinical symptoms that reappear regularly with the seasonal changes include lethargy, difficulty concentrating, depression, negative thoughts, elevated cravings for carbohydrates with corresponding overeating and weight gain, hypersomnia (excessive sleepiness), tiredness in the morning, diminished libido, and decreased social interaction. Patients typically become more anxious by the end of the summer as they anticipate the coming months, during which time less sunlight is present and their symptoms return. Clinical experience with patients reveals that they may have other mental problems as well, such as substance abuse disorders, personality or anxiety disorders, which, as co-morbid factors, further exacerbate the degree of the SAD patient's symptoms.

Flaws and Lake[1] define SAD as, "a variant of bipolar disorder characterized by cyclic manic, depressive or mixed mood states that are somehow triggered by external clues to changing seasons, including principally, increased or decreased day length. Individuals with SAD tend to become depressed during the autumn months and manic during the springtime." This is a complicated disorder that may accompany many severe illnesses, such as cardiovascular and endocrine disease and for which a patient should seek qualified professional help. Seasonal Affective Disorder does however, respond well to treatment with Oriental medicine.

My personal approach is to use acupuncture, herbs, and lifestyle modifications to address the disorder. While there is a core group of symptoms that patients share, each patient has their own medical history and clinical manifestations, mental or physical illnesses. If we treat the pattern that emerges, that is, differentiate and individualize the treatment, the best results are obtained.

There are many acupuncture points from which to choose to construct a treatment but in this chapter I will list some of my preferred points, their physiological energetics, and corresponding needle techniques. However, before selecting points, there are some general guidelines that can help structure the treatments:

- Keep treatments simple by addressing the root of the disorder instead of treating symptoms.
- Begin treatment at any point, however, the summer is ideal. By doing so, there is a good chance that the practitioner can break up the cyclic pattern of symptoms so that they are reduced or even eliminated before the problematic seasons arrive.
- Treat the patient one to two times a week depending upon which interval works best for them and in light of the degree of their symptoms.

Personally, I have found the primary point in the treatment of Seasonal Affective Disorder to be *yin tang*. *Yin tang* is located at the glabella, between the medial ends of the two eyebrows (see Fig. 13.**1**). Deep and posterior to the pituitary gland, at the base of the hypophysisis, lies the pineal gland, which responds to light and seasonal changes. When light levels are low the pineal gland secretes melatonin, a hormone that it also manufactures, which is involved in the regulation of sleep and mood disorders. Melatonin has the effect of sedating the body and promoting sleep. Hence, during seasons of low light the pineal gland constantly produces melatonin and a sleepy state is induced. By needling *yin tang*, the pineal gland can be stimulated such that both lethargy and depression are decreased.

Insert a thin needle such as a # 1 (36 g) needle through the point by threading it subcutaneously downward at a depth of 0.3 to 0.5 in. Moxa is contraindicated. If inserted painlessly and accurately,

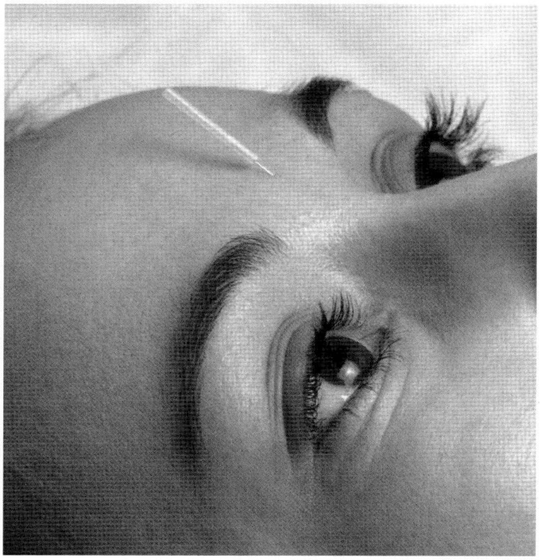

Fig. 13.1 Location of *yin tang* and needle method. Courtesy of Seirin Europe/3B Scientific, Hamburg, Germany.

patients love the effect of this point. Many patients have reported to me that they believe it has changed their mindset, alleviated depression, allowing them to be more relaxed yet invigorated. One of my patients referred to the feeling of this point as "heaven" as soon as I would needle it.

Liver 3 (*tai chong*) is known as a primary treatment point to redress the liver, which can easily be put out of balance due to its crucial role in the body as the mediator between the internal and external environments. As the *shu* (stream) point, earth point, and *yuan* (source) point, Liver 3 stabilizes, nourishes, and grounds the liver. It regulates the *zang fu* organs, quiets the mind, and makes the spirit peaceful. While many clinicians think of using Liver 3 for moving liver *qi* stagnation, it is actually better to adjust the relationship between the usual clinical scenarios of liver *yang* rising due to liver *yin* vacuity.

Liver 3 is a primary point for nourishing liver *yin*, and thereby moving stagnation by building *yin* versus simply moving stagnation alone, which is only appropriate for true excess conditions. I prefer threading Liver 3, 0.3 in proximally, or even connecting Liver 2 (*xin jian*), the sedation and fire point, to Liver 3 when signs of liver fire such as agitation, mania, insomnia, or signs of heat/fire are present. Locate both points in their standard location. The needle insertion in the direction of the channel is a tonification technique. Use a #1 (36 g) needle and treat bilaterally.

GV-20 (*bai hui*) is another important treatment point. As a Sea of Marrow it awakens and strengthens the brain. It pacifies the spirit, clears the mind, and stabilizes the will. It spreads liver *qi* and in cases of repletion, subdues the liver. Needle the point in a tonification direction, i. e., in this case anteriorly toward the face. If manic or fire symptoms predominate, needle the point in a sedation direction, that is, opposite the flow of the channel, downward towards the back of the head.

CV-4 (*guan yuan*), located 3 *cun* below the umbilicus along the midline of the body, is a central point to treat the kidney, liver, and spleen. It is referred to as the crossing point of the kidney, liver, and spleen channels on the abdomen, that is, it is analogous to SP-6 (*san yin jiao*), the group *luo* of the three-leg *yin*. It builds the kidney, adjusts the *qi*, builds blood and strengthens the foundation of the body. Puncture perpendicularly 0.5 to 1.2 in with a fine #1 (36 g), 1.5 in needle and obtain a mild stimulus. Moxa is also applicable for long amounts of time and frequent use as long as there are no signs of *yin* vacuity with heat/fire or excess heat.

Kidney 3 (*tai xi*) is another excellent point to include in the treatment of Seasonal Affective Disorder. Kidney 3, like Liver 3, is the source point of the channel and like all source points is useful in the treatment of chronic disorders and those that can benefit from accessing the pre-natal *jing* of that channel. Kidney 3 is also the *shu* (stream) point and earth point of the kidney channel, thereby balancing both kidney *yin* and *yang*.

According to the Chinese doctors I studied with in Beijing, Kidney 3 has four major functions—it tonifies kidney *qi* (i. e., the *yin* and *yang*) and tonifies source *qi*, blood, and essence. They also maintained that KI-3 is better than SP-6 to tonify *yin* and water while SP-6 is better for *yin* and dampness. Kidney 3 replenishes kidney *yin* when it is vacant, especially when there is a hyperactivity of liver fire. Kidney 3 strengthens the brain and willpower, the lack of which is a vacuity manifesting as depression.

The standard Chinese location of KI-3 is in the depression between the medial malleolus and tendo calcaneus, level with the tip of the medial malleolus. If selecting this location, puncture perpendicularly with a #1 (36 g) 1 in needle, insert shallowly, and obtain a mild stimulus to tonify kidney *yin*. A sensation radiating to the bottom of the foot is useful. Moxa is applicable. I prefer to needle the Japanese location of the point, which is identical to the Chinese location of KI-5. This point is called Japanese KI-3. It is defined as 1 *cun* directly below Chinese KI-3, in the depression anterior and superior to the medial side of the tuberosity of the calcaneum level with KI-6. Using a #1 (36 g) 1 in needle, puncture the point 0.3 to 0.5 in subcutaneously upward toward the Chinese location. If you prefer you can palpate both the Chinese and Japanese locations and select the point that is the most tender. Needle bilaterally. See Figure 13.**2a**, and **b** for the locations of both points.

While there are certainly more points that could be chosen to treat Seasonal Affective Disorder, this prescription of *yin tang*, LR-3 (*tai chong*), GV-20 (*bai hui*), CV-4 (*guan yuan*), and KI-3 (*tai xi*) is a simple model that works well and brings quick and immediate relief to the distressed patient. Herbal advice is outside the scope of this chapter because the person's entire presentation must be taken into account, but herbal therapy is valuable to treatment because it is biological supplementation. Below is a list of useful behavioral habits that the patient is encouraged to follow, which can augment the treatment.

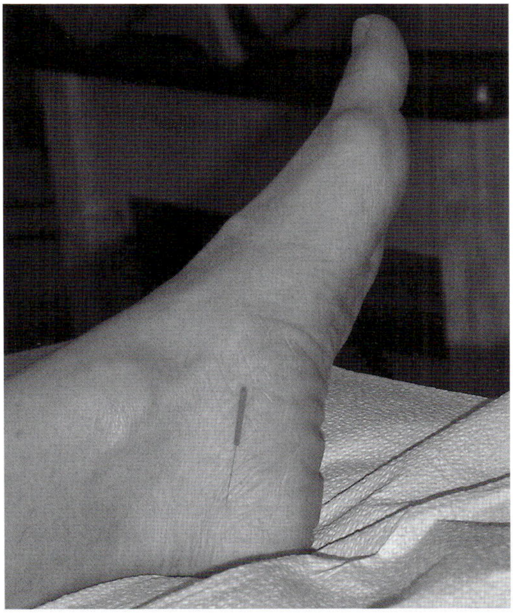

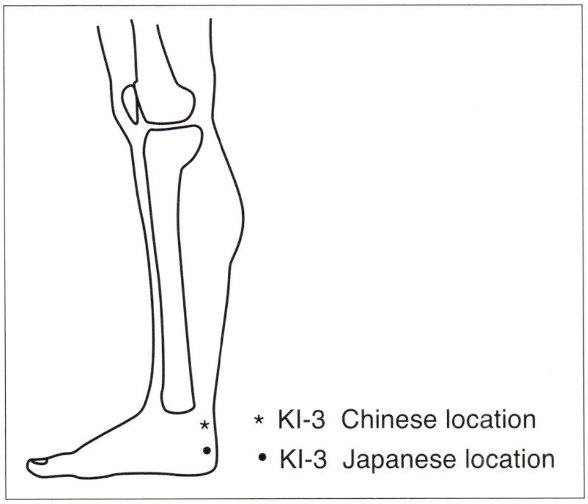

Fig. 13.**2a, b** Point locations of KI-3 (*tai xi*).

Advice for Patients with Seasonal Affective Disorder

- With Seasonal Affective Disorder one may crave carbohydrates in the form of starches and sweets. If needed, consume small amounts of breads, pastas, and pastries made of whole grains instead of white flour. Add more protein to the diet such as nuts, lean meat, fish, and small amounts of fat from cheeses or other sources, some fresh fruit, and plenty of cooked leafy vegetables, whole grains, and baked vegetables such as yams or baked potatoes.
- Exercise regularly by walking vigorously for 20 minutes, 5 to 7 days per week, in the morning or when there is the most sunlight.
- Work with lots of light by the windows to allow exposure to natural light and use full spectrum lighting in the house or workplace.
- Avoid overeating or gaining weight. Both will make the patient more tired and more sensitive and depressed.
- Try to go to bed earlier and get up earlier when there are more daylight hours. Avoid naps during the day that can interfere with sleep in the evening.
- Think positive, happy thoughts. Try not to worry or be fearful. Enjoy the warmth of family, friends, or any activity that brings "fire" to your life. Cultivate joy in your life.

Reference

1. Flaws B, Lake J. *Chinese Medical Psychiatry, a Textbook and Clinical Manual*. Boulder, CO: Blue Poppy Press; 2001:449.

14 A Simplified Approach to the Treatment of Scars

The treatment of scars has an historical base in Oriental medicine. Often, the treatment of scars can be the key to the successful resolution of chronic, persistent, and intractable conditions. All scars are inherently a malformation in normal cellular skin. They are matrices of collagen, blood vessels, and sometimes, foreign objects or toxins that have been deposited in a disorderly fashion. This constitutes the scarred tissue.

The way a scar develops depends on many factors. The most common factors tend to be the nature and severity of the original injury, the surgeon's skill or method of treatment, if any, that the scar received, how the person's body heals, the blood supply to the area, the direction of scar formation, and the color of one's skin.

According to Oriental medicine, essentially, scars can be viewed as "potential" organ-channel disturbances, that is, as potential physical or energetic disturbances of a channel precipitated by the trauma induced to the tissues. The disruption in energy flow in the skin, muscles, and underlying channels can then cause organic or energetic pathology of the local affected areas, internal and external channel pathways, corresponding *zang fu* organs and even distal sites.

Not all scars cause problems. Many are only superficial, or have healed such that the energy flow of the body is not affected. In general, factors such as scar size, abnormal coloration, lumpiness, and sensations associated with the scar, such as numbness, tingling, itchiness, heat, cold, achiness, and tendon/muscle restriction, indicate that the scar may need treating. Ultimately however, palpation of the discrete borders of the scar is the test to determine its clinical significance.

To evaluate the effects of scar tissue in relation to bodily health, first perform the scar evaluation described below:

1. Ask the patient if they have any scars. Remind them of possible scars from surgeries, injuries, and even vaccinations. Scars that are especially significant are found on the face, neck, scalp, back, and abdomen because of the major channels that traverse them.
2. Next, with your index finger, palpate all around the borders of the scar, at each place where your finger will fit. Press the tissue at about a 45° angle towards the scar at a moderate depth (about 0.5 in). If any area of the scar is tender, it may indicate *qi* and/or blood stagnation, *qi* and/or blood vacuity, or the accumulation of phlegm (calcification). Without the need to arrive precisely at a diagnosis, what is significant about the scar is the tenderness or pain at the affected area. This needs to be resolved since the lack of free-flowingness of energy may have significant effects on local and/or distal organs or sites.

There are numerous ways to treat scars. For convenience, the most common are described in Table **14.1**. More information on scar treatment may be found in *The Art of Palpatory Diagnosis in Oriental Medicine*.[1]

Before proceeding to treat with any modality, the following guidelines, cautions, and contraindications must be kept in mind:

- Do not treat scars that are still healing (less than a month old) to decrease the risk of infecting the scar.
- Observe clean needle technique so as not to infect the scar. Carefully treat scars in the elderly, diabetic patients, cancer patients, and those with neurological disorders or a weak constitution.
- Initially, only treat two tender areas of the scar until you can evaluate the effectiveness of scar treatment on the patient. In re-equilibrating energy in a scar, blocked energy may be released, leading to energy surges that the patient may perceive as a problem. For example, treating a scar on the gall bladder channel may release energy that goes to the head and produces a headache as the energy in the channel becomes unblocked.

Method	Instructions
External liniments	The application of external liniments and other products can aid in scar healing and reduce the imperfect formation of the epidermis. For convenience, liniments can be applied before bedtime so they have the chance to work for a relatively long period overnight. Useful liniments and their energetics include the following: *Zheng Gu Shui*—the deepest penetrating of all the Chinese liniments, it penetrates to the bone. It moves blood stasis, promotes healing via improved circulation, and stops pain Vitamin E (d-alpha tocopherol—don't use synthetic vitamin E designated by "acetate"). Vitamin E reduces superficial scarring and promotes normal tissue re-growth Aloe vera reduces scar formation, inflammation and swelling, and improves wound-healing capacity *Ching Wan Hung* promotes new tissue growth, reduces scarring and inflammation, and fights bacteria *Wan Hua* Oil activates blood stagnation and swelling caused by trauma
Needles	Before needling, palpate around the border of the scar and find the two most painful places. After swabbing those points with alcohol, insert a #1 (36 g) 30 mm (1 in) Seirin needle transversely (subcutaneously) underneath the scar to a depth of about 0.5 in. I prefer to use the thinnest needles to re-establish subtly even the minutest energetic pathways. However, if the scar is dense, thick, and fibrous a #3 or #5 gauge needle may be used so as not to bend or break the needle. Do not obtain *de qi* sensation, nor tonify nor disperse, but rather move the needle underneath the scar, then pull out and then repeat insertion two to three times. What the needle is used for is to break up obstruction mechanically if present or to stimulate the affected area. Stop at that depth or when resistance is felt. Retain the needles 5 to 10 minutes and remove. Continue this style of treatment during patient visits until no tender spots remain, at which point the scar is considered non-problematic. See Figure 14.**1a** and **b** for an illustrations of needle placement
Intradermal needles	In place of acupuncture needles, intradermal needles may be substituted. Follow the preliminary procedure as described under "Needles" above, which is to use palpation as the method to determine which two points to treat. Then using tweezers or forceps for support, insert a 0.6 mm Spinex intradermal needle under the scar. Secure the intradermal with Dermicel tape. Intradermals may be retained for take-home therapy or used in the office. However, do not retain intradermal needles on areas where clothing or physical activity may bend or displace them, i.e., at the wrist level, ankles, etc. Observe all standard precautions for the use of intradermals such as number of days to retain, avoiding getting wet, etc.
Tiger thermie warmer	The tiger thermie warmer is one of the most effective methods of scar treatment because it can be used to treat the entire scar versus two discrete points at a time as in needling. The tiger thermie warmer is a unique instrument that not only confers the therapeutic benefits of moxa directly onto the skin for penetration, but also simultaneously breaks up physical or energetic tension through the method of massage application with the tool. To appreciate and evaluate the effectiveness of the tiger thermie warmer, first palpate the borders of the scar looking for areas of tenderness. Travel around the borders of the scar with the tiger thermie warmer using light pressure on each discrete point. Move from point to point. Frequently check the temperature of the tiger thermie warmer to avoid burning the patient's skin. Apply the moxa to the scar borders for 1.5–3 minutes: the longer time for a larger scar. Following the moxa therapy, re-palpate the scar borders—there should be a reduction in tenderness. The area should get slightly pink and the patient should enjoy the relaxing treatment. Continue this approach in the office or instruct patients how to treat themselves daily or when convenient until no more tender spots remain

Table 14.**1** Methods of scar treatment

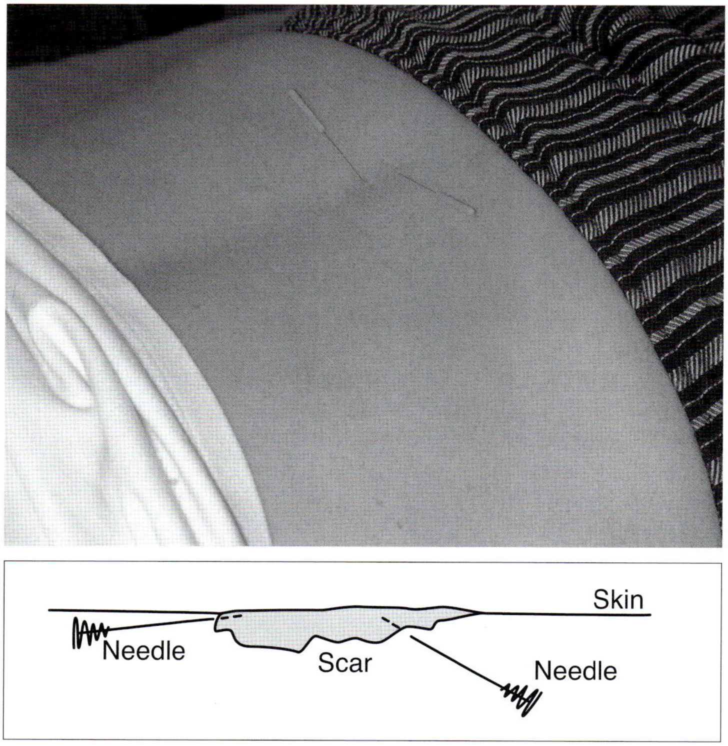

Fig. 14.**1a, b** How to needle a scar.

In conclusion, the treatment of scars with Oriental medicine is significant, simple, and successful, not just for the local alleviation of *qi* and blood stasis or vacuity, but concomitantly for its distal effects on channel pathways, patient perception and the overall health of the person. Figure 14.**1a** and **b** demonstrates the needling of scar tissue.

Reference

1. Gardner-Abbate S. *The Art of Palpatory Diagnosis in Oriental Medicine*. London: Churchill Livingstone; 2001.

15 Shoulder Problems: A Quick and Comprehensive Approach

Shoulder pain is a common problem. In terms of its success rate with acupuncture, it is one of the easier musculoskeletal disorders to treat. This chapter presents four treatment options that I commonly choose from, all which are effective and easy to execute. The practitioner is encouraged to review and select those that he/she prefers and that can best help the patient.

First, regardless of the treatment selected, have the patient explain the etiology of the problem, its duration, intensity, what makes it better or worse, and other relevant characteristics. Determine the range of motion the patient has by having them move their arm and shoulder in all the normal movements (rotation [lateral and medial], abduction, adduction, flexion, and extension), and evaluate the type of impaired mobility they have.

■ Auricular Acupuncture

Personally, I typically choose ear massage and treatment as my first and most successful therapeutic modality because of my affinity for auricular medicine and its proven effectiveness.

In the ear, locate the shoulder point if the problem is musculoskeletal or the shoulder joint point if the problem is confined to the joint. Vigorously rub the chosen ear point between your thumb and index finger. Do this with the patient seated or standing. Let the patient know they will feel a very strong sensation elicited by the rubbing. Perform this step for 15 to 30 seconds. The stimulus will be very intense and the patient may grimace or tell you it is painful. After this time span, have the patient make the shoulder movements that were performed earlier. In most cases, if your ear point location was accurate, you achieved the desired stimulus (i. e., strong sensation and/or heat), and the patient can tolerate it, there will be 50–100% improvement in the shoulder. If this technique has been effective, but you feel the shoulder needs further reinforcement, you can affix a Magrain pellet or an ear seed to the point so that the patient can retain it for about three days. Instruct them to rub it gently three to five times a day for about 3 to 5 seconds and at the same time to mobilize the affected shoulder.

If their shoulder problem is along the large intestine channel, select the shoulder point on the contralateral (opposite) side of the patient's shoulder pain. The reason for treating the opposite side is that the large intestine's divergent channel exits at LI-15 (*jian yu*) and so the point on the opposite side will treat the shoulder pain. If the pain is more posterior, i. e., along the scalene muscles or in the Gall Bladder 21 (*jian jing*) area, select the ear point on the same side as the patient's shoulder problem. See Figure 15.**1** for the location of these points.

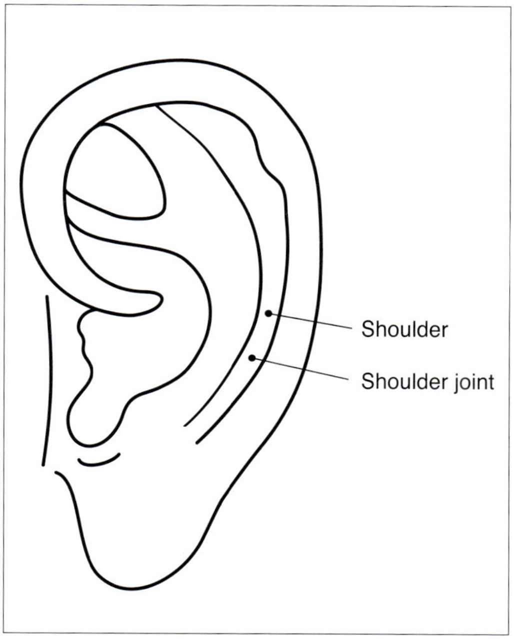

Fig. 15.**1** The shoulder and shoulder joint ear points.

Needle LU-7

Another interesting treatment of shoulder pain, especially if it appears anterior to the acromioclavicular joint, is to treat the lung. Remember the lung channel internally transverses the shoulder area where it exits at LU-1 (*zhong fu*). With the patient reclining, needle LU-7 (*lie que*) transversely 0.5 – 1.0 in proximally (towards the shoulder). Do this unilaterally on the side of the affected shoulder problem. In this instance you are using Lung 7 as a longitudinal *luo*, that is, as a connecting vessel on the lung channel, to send a stimulus to the lung organ/channel complex.

After attaining *de qi*, use a vigorous dispersion technique. I prefer speed and large amplitude for 5 to 10 seconds. The patient should feel the *qi* go strongly up the arm. Then remove the needle and have the patient mobilize the affected shoulder and evaluate therapeutic success. There can be substantial improvement.

Tuina and/or Needles

If the problem is directly at the shoulder joint, precisely at LI-15 (*jian yu*), two options are possible—*tuina* and needles. With the patient seated, vigorously rub LI-15 with a deep and rapid manipulation. The Chinese I studied *tuina* with in Beijing say to rub this point 200 times in this manner. My experience is that most American patients cannot tolerate such a strong sensation for that length of time nor can all practitioners execute this technique. So looking at the patient, I monitor how the treatment is affecting them and rub with a deep, precise, vigorous motion as long as I can. This may be only 20 seconds. Again this technique is extremely strong, but works very fast and is unequivocally efficacious for this type of shoulder pain. It is similar to the auricular treatment in that massage is used. It is ideal for frozen shoulder.

You may choose to needle this point also. The point can be needled perpendicularly into the joint, or obliquely down the arm. Choose a perpendicular insertion if it is a joint problem or an oblique insertion if upper arm muscles are involved. Insert the needle 1.0 to 1.5 in perpendicularly, or obliquely and subcutaneously down the arm to the same depth and disperse the point. Even though needling is unilateral, this is a powerful needle technique and has a strong bearing down sensation. I find that patients prefer the *tuina* to the needle technique for this differentiation of shoulder pain.

Threading

Finally, another classical Chinese option, is threading ST-38 (*tiao kou*) to BL-57 (*cheng shan*). Bladder 57 has the property of relaxing the muscle channels, and ST-38, close to ST-37 (*shang ju xu*), the inferior *he* (uniting) point of the large intestine, has an effect on the shoulder. In combination they assist in the treatment of shoulder pain.

Puncture ST-38 obliquely as you thread towards BL-57. Using a 2 to 3 in needle, unilaterally insert it to a depth of 1.0 to 1.5 in on the right leg since stomach/large intestine energetics are more right-sided as can be seen in the pulse system where the stomach and large intestine appear in the right pulse. Even though the depth of insertion is relatively deep, this should not be a painful insertion. Using an insertion tube, simply tap the needle into the epidermis and then slowly insert to achieve the through-and-through technique. When you are at the proper depth, keep manipulating the needle with a combined lift and thrust and wide amplitude technique. At this point, because you are deeply embedded in the musculature, the manipulation of the needle will feel heavy and sticky and this will produce a strong sensation in the leg. Let the patient know this. Manipulate the needle for a half a minute or so, then remove it and have the patient mobilize the shoulder. Often there is significant improvement. This technique can be used for arthritis of the shoulder as well as peripheral inflammation of the shoulder.

In conclusion, these are simple yet comprehensive treatment strategies that have known clinical efficacy in the treatment of shoulder pain. Only one needs to be used at a time. They work; the treatment is fast, and the results are long-lasting for the patient. As always these techniques are a testimony to the inter-relatedness of body systems and the sagacity of Oriental medicine.

■ Point Location Reminders

- LI-15: anteroinferior to the acromion, in the middle of the upper portion of the muscle deltoideus. When the arm is in full abduction, the point is in the anterior depression of the two depressions appearing at the anterior border of the acromioclavicular joint.
- LU-7: superior to the styloid process of the radius, 1.5 *cun* above the transverse crease of the wrist, in the depression on the styloid process of the radius.
- ST-38: 8 *cun* below ST-35 (*du bi*), 2 *cun* below ST-37 (*shang ju xu*), midway between ST-37 and ST-41 (*jie xi*).
- BL-57: directly below the belly of the muscle gastrocnemius, on the line connecting BL-40 (*wei zhong*) and tendo calcaneus, about 8 *cun* below BL-40.
- Shoulder ear point: located in the scapha, level with the crus of the helix.
- Shoulder joint ear point: located in the scapha, midway between the shoulder and the clavicle points.

16 Repetitive Motion Disorders

Repetitive motion syndrome is a malady that affects millions of people. Its clinical manifestations include numbness or tingling (with or without pain) in the forearm, wrist, hands, or fingers. Weakness in thumb abduction may be present as well as tendon inflammation and swelling. It may present unilaterally or bilaterally. It is named as such because its etiology is due to repetitive motions such as typing, computer work, or other labor involving repetitious motion or the overuse of the tendons.

Carpal tunnel syndrome is a painful wrist disorder caused by compression of the median nerve. It is commonly thought of as being caused by repetitive motion and sometimes it is. It is the leading compensable occupational illness, surpassing back injuries since 1990. However, a correct diagnosis of carpal tunnel syndrome requires adherence to strict electro-physiological data. Many of the studies that have supported the notion that carpal tunnel syndrome is a repetitive motion disorder have not used exact clinical data and have rarely included electro-diagnostic information.[1]

Carpal tunnel syndrome specifically, and repetitive motion syndrome in general, have always been viewed as being treated well with Oriental medicine, especially with acupuncture. Standard treatments revolve around treating points such as PC-7 (*da ling*), PC-9 (*zhong chong*), LI-11 (*qu chi*), TB-5 (*wai guan*), and LI-4 (*he gu*), which are local to the affected areas. Although this treatment is viable as well, my treatment approach is somewhat different and has yielded excellent clinical results for me. It is described below.

From an observational point of view, the problem of carpal tunnel syndrome and repetitive motion syndrome is confounded by the simultaneous presence of repetitive motions, the neurovascular compression of nerves coming from the shoulder area, and arterial compression. Painters, artists, computer technicians, cashiers, or assembly-line workers who type or perform repetitive motions of the wrist also develop a postural accommodation that leads to shoulder and neck tension.

When the shoulders slouch forward and the chest becomes slightly concave, abnormal compression of the subclavian artery or the axillary, and/or the brachial plexus may result. This compression produces a series of signs and symptoms such as pain and numbness in the distal extremities of the forearm, wrist, hands, and fingers, which is termed neurovascular compression. Patients with this problem typically have stiff neck, shoulders, and back, and often headaches. My typical treatment style revolves around alleviating the compression and removing the stagnation that manifests in the signs and symptoms of carpal tunnel and repetitive motion syndromes.

In my treatment repertoire, the most important point to alleviate the neurovascular and arterial compression is ST-12 (*que pen*). Stomach 12 is located in midpoint of the supraclavicular fossa 4 *cun* lateral to the *ren* channel. Treating it can loosen up the tissue and muscles of the supraclavicular fossa, which are tight or constrained due to posture, stress, or tension. Consider this point to be more of an area that encompasses the discrete point as well as about 1.5 to 1 in above it.

Stomach 12 is a highly underutilized point in many practitioners' repertoire of points. However, it possesses powerful and unique energetics, which account for its efficacy. Firstly, ST-12 is the point of intersection of many channels. It is the union of the stomach, small intestine, triple burner, and gall bladder channels. It is its unique anatomical position that accounts for its therapeutic usefulness. Anatomically it is directly above the supraclavicular portion of the brachial plexus. Its traditional indications center on cough, asthma, sore throat, and pain in the supraclavicular fossa, stiff neck, and neck spasms.

Even if the repetitive motion syndrome or the carpal tunnel syndrome is only one-sided, treat the point bilaterally. If needling is done for this treatment, the patient should recline in the lateral recumbent position (on their side). Gently insert a #1 gauge 30 mm needle perpendicularly 0.3 to 0.5 *cun* posterior to the sternocleidomastoid muscle. Note this is not the usual Chinese method of needling ST-12, which is perpendicularly downward, but rather a Japanese technique. Do not obtain *qi*, nor tonify, nor disperse; that is, do not manipulate, turn, lift, thrust, or use any other technique with the needle. See Figure 11.**2** in Chapter 11, which illustrates the regional anatomy as well as the needle placement for ST-12.

Needle with caution. Carefully monitor the angle and depth of insertion due to proximity to the apex of the lung so it is not in danger of being punctured. Retain the needle for 10 to 15 minutes and then reverse sides. Additionally, I add distal points along the channels that may be involved such as LI-1 (*shang yang*), LU-11 (*shao shang*), LI-11 (*qu chi*) and PC-9 (*zhong chong*). The *jing* (well) points can be needled perpendicularly 0.1 *cun* or bled by using a bleeding technique to remove the stasis and smooth the course of *qi* and blood in the channels. Obtain one to two drops of blood. Large Intestine 11 can be needled perpendicularly 1.0 to 1.5 in.

Moxibustion is an added modality that can be integrated into the treatment. Apply gentle moxa in the form of a moxa pole to ST-12 and LI-11 for approximately 3 minutes on each point until the patient reports radiating warmth. If massage is performed, gently massage the point for about 20 seconds on each side.

This treatment can be performed once a week for three to five treatments. At the end of this course of treatment the problem is usually alleviated. Additionally, I tend to augment the treatment with a generous application of the liniment *Zheng Gu Shui*, the best Chinese liniment for *qi* and blood stasis. Apply it along the course of the affected channels with a cotton ball. I recommend that the patient apply it to the same areas before going to bed every evening. Use caution not to get the liniments into mucous membranes or the eyes.

Lifestyle counseling should also be provided to eliminate these as etiological factors. The person should cultivate a sense of their posture, take frequent breaks from repetitive motions, obtain massage, do gentle neck exercises like rotations, and use ergonomically designed seating, wristpads, and keyboards if their use is indicated. Sometimes a vitamin B6 vacuity may account for improper neurological functioning and unless otherwise contraindicated, a good-quality multivitamin can assist in restoring and maintaining proper nerve functioning.

Reference

1. Kirschberg G, Fillingim R, Davis VP, Hogg F. Carpal tunnel syndrome: classic clinical symptoms and electrodiagnostic studies in poultry workers with hand, wrist, and forearm pain. *South Med J.* March 1994;87(3).

III Other Modalities—Treatment Tools Complementary to Acupuncture

17 Bleeding Techniques: Ancient Treatment for Acupuncture Physicians

An ancient Oriental treatment technique applicable for many conditions, but which the modern day practitioner may be hesitant to use in his/her treatment plans, is bloodletting. The reluctance to use this method could be due to the drawing of blood that can transmit blood-borne pathogens, or maybe there is some concern about causing the patient potential discomfort. However, bleeding is a specialized technique for specific conditions that can produce effective and dramatic results when the patient's condition is properly diagnosed and the bleeding method expertly executed and matched to the diagnosis. Bloodletting has four major therapeutic aims that are useful in the clinical arena. Let us review them:

1. It can invigorate the smooth flow of *qi* and blood, thereby augmenting and facilitating the free flow of the *qi* when it needs invigoration. An example of this is when a patient presents with a wiry pulse and mild feelings of distention that indicate liver *qi* stagnation and the *qi* simply needs to be moved.
2. It disperses *qi* and blood stasis as in the case of backache or spider veins caused by *qi* and blood stagnation.
3. It can drain excess heat and fire. Such excess includes pathogenic factors, for instance caused by an invasion of the lung by wind heat that produces a fever and very sore throat.
4. Finally, bleeding can bring down *yang* rising as in the variety of high blood pressure due to liver *yang* rising. Note: not all hypertension has this etiology and hence bloodletting is not suitable for those differentiations.

There are numerous clinical conditions that are suitable for treatment with bleeding that have the four differentiations listed above, and some of these are outlined later in Tables 17.**1** and 17.**2**.

The categories of acupuncture points that are the most common to bleed are those that have shallow depths of insertions such as ear acupuncture points, scalp points, and *jing* (well) points. Other points that can be bled are those whose energetics lend themselves to bleeding such as BL-40 (*wei zhong*), to release summer heat, the ear apex point for acute conjunctivitis, or local points for pathologies such as bruises or varicosities.

There are three types of bleeding techniques. The first is called the spot pricking or collateral (collateral = channel) pricking method. With this style of needling a discrete point or spot is bled such as a *jing* (well) point like LI-1 (*shang yang*) to relieve a toothache due to excess heat, or LU-11 (*shao shang*) to treat a sore throat due to excess heat.

The second method is called the clumping or area pricking method. With this approach pinprick motions are made on a relatively large point such as GV-14 (*da zhui*) to reduce excess heat in the lungs as in the case of pneumonia.

The last type of bleeding is called the pinching method. With this technique the point treated is pinched between the thumb and the index fingers and held while the practitioner punctures the point. This action isolates the point as well as promotes venous pooling, which facilitates bleeding. Bladder 2 (*zan zhu*) is a common point to pinch and bleed for sinus congestion or headache.

As effective as it, bleeding is contraindicated for certain conditions. One of the most important prohibitions is that it is not suitable for *yin* vacuity or false heat. Bleeding in this case can actually weaken the patient, as the heat is not real but is arising from vacuity.

In general, patients with diabetes, bleeding disorders such as hemophilia, or patients who may bleed easily such as those on blood thinners, should not be bled. Bleeding contraindications equally apply to patients who are extremely weakened, anemic, hypotensive, or pregnant. Depending upon the point treated, the patient can be bled either in a sitting position for bleeding a *jing* (well) point, or in a reclining position in order to pinch BL-2 for instance.

Points	Bleeding Method	Clinical Conditions
LU-11 (*shao shang*)	Spot pricking	Sore throat of the excess type, external heat invasions, tonsillitis, stuffiness and pain in the chest, asthmatic breathing, stomach ache, frontal shoulder pain
LI-1 (*shang yang*)	Spot pricking	Toothache, sore throat, nasal obstruction, seasonal allergies, tinnitus, frontal headache, stomach ache, shoulder pain
HT-9 (*shao chong*)	Spot pricking	Febrile diseases, stuffiness and pain in the chest, palpitations, angina pectoris, insomnia, headache, tinnitus, shoulder pain, back pain, heart attack
SI-1 (*shao ze*)	Spot pricking	Febrile diseases, breast disorders
BL-2 (*zan zhu*)	Pinching	Wind-heat in the eyes, acute conjunctivitis, sinus pressure and headache
BL-40 (*wei zhong*)	Pinching	Back pain, acute lumbar sprain, multiple furuncles and swelling, sunstroke, leg pain
BL-67 (*zhi yin*)	Spot pricking	Back pain along the bladder channel
PC-3 (*qu ze*)	Spot pricking	Febrile disease, acute vomiting
PC-9 (*zhong chong*)	Spot pricking	Coma, unconsciousness, stuffiness and pain in the chest, palpitations, angina, insomnia, stomach problems, pain in the liver region
TB-1 (*guan chong*)	Spot pricking	Tinnitus, migraines, sore throat, shoulder pain, back pain, pain in the chest and hypochondriac region, hepatic distending pain
LR-1 (*da dun*)	Spot pricking	Irritability, red eyes, high blood pressure, liver headaches (at the vertex), genital pain
GV-4 (*ming men*)	Pinching	Lumbago
GV-14 (*da zhui*) and its *Huatoujiajis*	Pinching	Excess lung heat, pneumonia, febrile disease
Extra points *Yin tang*	Pinching	Headache, cerebral infarction
Tai yang	Pinching	Headache at the temple area
Ear apex (in the ear)	Pinching	High blood pressure, acute conjunctivitis, spasms, high fever caused by toxicity, wind, heat, liver *yang* rising
Jin jin and *yu ye* (veins under the tongue)	Pinching	Pernicious vomiting, morning sickness, aphasia
Shi xuan (tips of fingers)	Spot pricking	Coma, epilepsy, infantile convulsion, convulsion, sunstroke

Table 17.**1** Points, bleeding method, and clinical conditions

Points	Bleeding Method	Clinical Conditions
Si feng (midpoint of interphalangeal joints of all fingers except thumb)	Spot pricking	Digestive disorders in children (prick when purple)
Ba xie (junction of margin of webs of fingers)	Spot pricking	Spasm and contracture of the fingers (pathologic fluid may come out)
Other		
Spider veins	Spot pricking	On the face for sinus congestion
Local points	Spot pricking	As in herpes zoster (shingles): for herpes above the waist use LU-11 and for herpes below the waist use SP-1; sprains on chest wall
Jing (well) points	Spot pricking	In general for resuscitation, coma apoplexy, mental disorders, sore throat, toothache, chest fullness. Specifically see *jing* (well) points listed above
Luo points	Clumping method	Swollen ankles, for acute local swelling
Hypertension groove in the ear	Pinching	High blood pressure due to liver *yang* rising
Point combinations		
LI-4 (*he gu*), LI-11 (*qu chi*)	Pinching or clumping method	Numbness
ST-36 (*zu san li*), GV-26 (*shui gou*), PC-3 (*qu ze*), BL-40 (*wei zhong*), PC-6 (*nei guan*)	Clumping	Hypertension
BL-40 (*wei zhong*), LU-5 (*chi ze*), ST-44 (*nei ting*), PC-3 (*qu ze*)	Spot pricking or pinching	Sunstroke, food poisoning, acute gastroenteritis
GB-14 (*yang bai*), ST-4 (*di cang*), ST-6 (*jia che*), SI-18 (*quan liao*)	Clumping or pinching	Facial paralysis
GV-14 (*da zhui*), BL-12 (*feng men*), BL-15 (*xin shu*), BL-17 (*ge shu*), BL-20 (*pi shu*)	Clumping or pinching	Relapsing urticaria
GV-2 (*yao shu*), BL-32 (*ci liao*), BL-25 (*da chang shu*)	Clumping	Acute hemorrhoids
GV-20 (*bai hui*) and *a-shi* points	Clumping	Press GV-20 and bleed *a-shi* points for stiff neck
LI-11 (*qu chi*), L-4 (*he gu*), SP-6 (*san yin jiao*), LR-2 (*sing xian*), ST-44 (*nei ting*)	Clumping or pinching	Eczema
LR-5 (*li gou*), ST-40 (*feng long*), BL-13 (*fei shu*), GV-14 (*da zhui*)	Spot pricking	Damp heat eczema
BL-17 (*ge shu*), BL-20 (*pi shu*), ST-36 (*zu san li*)	Clumping or pinching	Skin problems due to wind dryness (blood vacuity)

Table 17.**1** Points, bleeding method, and clinical conditions (cont.)

Prior to bleeding the practitioner should have all of the required treatment tools within the work area. Next, hands are washed and a clean field is established with paper towels or professional toweling, upon which are placed dry sterile cotton balls, alcohol preps, tight-fitting protective gloves, and the bleeding tool of choice. Off the field have an open biohazard sharps container, a biohazard trash container, extra gloves, and goggles and facemask in the event of excessive bleeding. Don a double pair of tight fitting gloves to guard against the transmission of infectious blood-borne pathogens. As always, the point to be bled is swabbed with 70% isopropyl alcohol and allowed to dry naturally.

Bleeding tools include the regular acupuncture or filiform needle, a medical lancet, the *shoni-shin* needle (Japanese pediatric needle), the traditional three-edge needle, or the plum blossom needle (seven-star or cutaneous needle). Use a #28 or #30 g, 15-mm acupuncture needle.

If using the spot pricking or pinching method, the discomfort of bleeding can virtually be eliminated by a rapid speed of insertion to the desired shallow depth of about 0.05 to 0.1 *cun*. Elicit one to two drops of blood (some practitioners say up to ten) by squeezing the point. Absorb the blood with sterile cotton and dispose of the cotton in the biohazard trash container along with the used gloves. If there is so much blood in the cotton ball such that it can be wrung out (which should not be the case in proper bleeding technique), it must be disposed of in a biohazard unit. Immediately dispose of the bleeding tool if it is not reusable in the sharps container after pricking the point. Place a Band-Aid (sticking plaster) on most points that are bled (i.e., distal *jing* [well] points) to allow them to heal and to prevent infection and then wash your hands.

Clinical Notes

1. Points need only be needled unilaterally, generally on the affected side of the body, for instance for right-sided toothache of the lower right quadrant, bleed the right side LI-1 point (*shang yang*), which treats this type of toothache. If side is not pertinent, use the side corresponding to the pulse system. For instance, if the person has left-sided temple pain along the gall bladder channel, the chosen point such GB-44 (*zu qiao yin*) can be treated because the gall bladder is represented in pulse systems on the left pulse. Bilateral needling is unnecessary, may cause added discomfort, and does not contribute further to the results. Clinical trail and error shows that when the point is bled bilaterally, less blood is elicited from the side that does not need bleeding.
2. Lancets are excellent to use to bleed *jing* (well) points but in general are too big and jarring for body acupuncture points.
3. Remember, bleeding is not appropriate for *yin* vacuity heat.
4. The application of the Chinese herbal liniment *Zheng Gu Shui* to an area on which the plum blossom needle is used helps with any bruising or extravasations caused by the plum blossom and further aids in promoting *qi* and blood flow and resolving blood stasis.
5. Do not treat every little spider vein that is a result of age, gravity, or standing too much on one's feet. They tend to reoccur because the etiology is not addressed. However, spider veins due to trauma are treated well with bleeding.

The frequency of bleeding is contingent upon the patient's medical condition. If the patient has an excess heat condition such as tonsillitis, bleeding can be performed once a day until the symptoms abate. If the patient has a blood stasis condition bleeding can be done one to two times per week.

Table 17.**1** summarizes common points amenable to bleeding, the style of bleeding technique to use, and the clinical conditions related to the points that are bled. Table 17.**2** correlates the clinical results of bleeding with specific modalities.

Condition	Modality	Result
Trauma to hip/buttocks	Plum blossom	Improvement by 90 – 100 %
Spider veins	Plum blossom	Reduction in appearance
Pain in temples	Lancet GB - 44 (*zu giao yin*)/ TB - 17 (*yi feng*)	Pain decreased by 70 %
Hip/sciatic pain	Lancet GB - 44 (*zu giao yin*)	Pain decreased by 30 %
Coughing, chest tightness, restlessness	Bleeding LU - 1 (*zhong fu*)/ LR - 1 (*da dun*)	Chest and throat pain relieved
Severe sore throat	Lancet LU - 11 (*qu chi*)	60 % improvement
Rash, canker sore, acne	Needle BL - 40 (*wei zhong*)	Rash and fever decreased
Excess heat: migraines, anger, violent etc.	Needle HT - 9 (*shao chong*)	Calmer, headache decreased
Allergy symptoms, itchy eyes etc.	Needle LI - 11 (*shang yang*)	Immediate relief
Shoulder pain	Lancet LI - 1 (*zan zhu*)	100 % reduction in pain, 80 % improvement in range of motion
Neck and scapular pain	Needle SI - 1	35 – 40 % reduction in pain
Allergy headache	Needle BL - 2	Instant relief
Swollen index finger	Bleed finger point in the ear	Quick relief of pain and swelling
Irritability, nausea, red eyes	Lancet LR - 1 (*da dun*)	Immediately calm, 80 % reduction in eye redness the next day
Shoulder pain	Needle SI - 1 (*shao ze*)	70 – 80 % improvement in range of motion

Table 17.**2** Bleeding results and corresponding modalities for specific clinical conditions

18 Liniments, Sprays, and Powders

Chinese first aid liniments are an easy and effective first choice or method of augmentation to treat a variety of musculoskeletal disorders. These common clinical complaints can be addressed by applying liniments in the clinical setting and by teaching the patients how to use them appropriately at home. While there are other categories of Chinese herbal products that the practitioner can teach his/her patients to use, such as the use of common digestive and respiratory herbs, these areas require a deeper understanding of Chinese diagnosis that exceed the scope of this chapter.

The Oriental medical practitioner is encouraged to instruct patients in the use of first aid liniments. Even thought they are easy to learn, always provide written instructions to the patient on how to use each one for his/her own safety, and for proper medico-legal documentation. For clinician convenience, Table 18.**1** summarizes the use of the most popular Chinese liniments, sprays, and powders, and they are discussed below. Forms to write out prescriptions for each of these products are provided in the Appendix and may be reproduced to give to patients.

Chinese liniments, derived in Chinese history largely from the branch of medicine called "Hit Medicine" (or medications developed from *kung fu* and battle injuries), are a very useful method of treatment largely for musculoskeletal disorders. Over the years, many liniments have been produced and are part of the Chinese pharmacopoeia. The ones I use extensively in my clinical practice

Liniment	Energetics	Clinical Use	Special Notes/i.e., Contraindications
1. *Zheng Gu Shui* (liquid)	Hot energetically; penetrates to bone level; promotes osteoblast production, promotes healing of fractures, disperses blood and fluid stagnation; invigorates *qi* and blood, stops pain, relaxes tendons and muscles. Composed of herbs that move blood, open to the exterior	Bone spurs, headache, blood stasis, pain of neck, back, ankles, shoulders, arthritic conditions, bruises	Apply generously with cotton ball or spray. Do not use on conditions of inflammation with heat. Avoid mucous membranes. Do not heat up or cover; flammable; stains clothes. Do not use with *tuina*. Do not apply to open wounds. Do not cover up tightly
2. Woodlock Oil (liquid)	Similar to Regal Oil (*Kwan Loong*); more "body" to oil	Arthritis, muscle tension	For external use only. Do not use with *tuina*. Avoid contact with eyes. Do not apply to wounds or damaged skin or bandage tightly. Do not use under age of 2—may cause burns
3. Regal Oil (*Kwan Loong*) (liquid)	Similar to White Flower; cool energetically	Arthritis, muscle aches	For external use. Avoid contact with eyes
4. White Flower Oil (liquid)	Relieves itching, stops swelling, reduces inflammation; cool energetically	Headache, bites, arthritis, neuralgia	Mostly for external use. Avoid contact with eyes

Table 18.**1** First aid liniments, sprays, and powders

Liniment	Energetics	Clinical Use	Special Notes/i.e., Contraindications
5. *Po Sum On* Oil (liquid)	Warm energetically; invigorates blood, dispels cold	Wind-cold aches, blood stagnation injury, topically for toothache and sore throat, apply externally to chest for chest cough	Avoid eyes and open wounds, FLAMMABLE, apply liberally, frequently
6. *Wan Hua* Oil (liquid)	Warm energetically; promotes blood circulation, relieves pain, transforms stagnation, relaxes sinews and tendons	Burns, trauma, bleeding, "stricken, fallen, shocken, and twisten conditions"	Use on burn or cut i.e., open wounds several times a day
7. *Yunnan Pai Yao* (powder)	Disperses stagnant blood, stops bleeding, invigorates blood, stops pain. Main ingredient—raw pseudo ginseng	Traumatic bleeding and swelling, hot skin infections, bleeding ulcers, insect bites, excessive menstrual cramps and bleeding	Use on open wounds or cuts and apply pressure until bleeding stops. For internal and external use. Internally for ulcers, menstrual cramps. For serious wounds or bleeding take red pill
8. Plaster for bruises and analgesic	Promotes circulation of blood, stimulates healing, stops pain, cooling	Sprains, bruises, fractures, swelling, neuralgia, arthritis, rheumatism, muscle tenderness, muscle strain, musculoskeletal pain due to wind	Apply to clean, dry, hair-free skin; retain a few days. Do not apply to lower abdomen or low back area during pregnancy. Do not use under 2 years of age. Avoid contact with eyes. Do not apply to wounds or damaged skin. Do not apply tightly
9. Spray moxa	Penetrates to the channel level, moves *qi* and blood, tonifies *yang*	Joint pain, muscle strain, bruises, swelling, fractures	Spray on affected area—note: it goes on cold so prepare patient by letting know as it may cause contraction. Apply *Zheng Gu Shui* first and then spray moxa, or apply TDP lamp over area. Needs heat to activate it. *Zheng Gu Shui* does this. Do not use during pregnancy
10. *Ching Wan Hung* (ointment)	Promotes circulation of *qi* or blood, cools heat, stops pain immediately, promotes tissue growth, reduces swelling and blistering, prevents infection, deputrifies, acts as a bactericide	Skin diseases, bedsores, skin cancers, hemorrhoids, sunburn, heat rash, for large area deep burns and scalds caused by boiling water, oil, fire, steam, molten steel or radioactive/chemical substances	Cover with bandage; clean and change daily; stains

Notes:
- Most liniments will stain clothes. Stain can be removed with rubbing alcohol.
- With all liniments, avoid eyes and mucous membranes. Generally avoid open wounds.
- Discontinue if allergic skin reaction occurs.
- Some of these can be taken internally. See standard herbal texts on method and amount.
- Keep these and all drugs out of the reach of children. In case of accidnetal ingestion, seek professional assistance of contact a poison control center immediately.

Table 18.**1** First aid liniments, sprays, and powders (cont.)

are described below and all can be safely used on patients as well as taught to them so they can use them as first aid remedies. Some of the products are liquids (called liniments), some are powders, ointments, or spray medium.

Zheng Gu Shui

Zheng Gu Shui is my liniment of choice because it has a broad range of clinical applications and can be used for many first aid situations. Energetically, on a continuum of cold to hot, *Zheng Gu Shui* is energetically the hottest of the Chinese liniments. By virtue of this *yang* function, it has the deepest penetrating power and is able to penetrate through the skin, muscle and channel layer all the way to the bone. When it reaches the bone it promotes the healing of fractures by stimulating osteoblast production. It can disperse blood and fluid stagnation, invigorate *qi* and blood, stop pain, and relax tendons and muscles. It is composed of herbs that move the blood and open to the exterior.

As a result of these properties, *Zheng Gu Shui* can treat bone spurs, cases of blood stasis such as bruises, and is excellent for musculoskeletal pain of the neck, back, ankles, elbows, knees, and any arthritic condition not characterized by heat or inflammation.

With a cotton ball, generously apply *Zheng Gu Shui* to the affected area. Do not use on conditions characterized by heat manifestations such as fever, swellings hot to the touch, or areas that are red or inflamed. Keep away from mucous membranes of the eyes, nose, mouth, and genital regions. Do not warm the liniment up. Do not cover the liniment that has been applied to the skin with gauze or Band-Aids (sticking plasters) as the captured heat can cause a serious burn. Do not use with massage or *tuina*, as the heat of the liniment and the heat of friction will also cause irritation. Do not apply to open wounds. *Zheng Gu Shui* will stain clothes.

Woodlock Oil

Woodlock Oil is another Chinese liniment that is very similar to Regal Oil. It is an amber-colored liniment, with more body than the clear Regal Oil, and is a warm liniment energetically.

While Regal Oil is known as an arthritis liniment, clinically, patients with osteoarthritis prefer Woodlock Oil because of its warm versus cooling nature, and those with rheumatoid arthritis prefer Regal Oil. Woodlock Oil is also a liniment for external use only. Do not use with *tuina* or massage because its warmth combined with the friction can cause irritation. Avoid contact with mucous membranes. Do not apply to wounds or damaged skin. Bandage lightly. Do not use on children as it may cause burns.

Regal Oil (*Kwan Loong*)

Regal oil is a clear, colorless, cool liquid. It is good for muscular aches and rheumatoid arthritis. It also for external use only. Avoid contact with mucous membranes.

White Flower Oil

White Flower Oil is a clear, colorless, cool liniment. It is one of the most common and well-known Chinese liniments because of its broad range of uses. It comes in different size bottles that look like little perfume bottles.

Energetically White Flower Oil is cooling; hence it relieves itching, stops swelling and inflammation. It is good for headaches, insect bites, rheumatoid arthritis, and neuralgia. It is mostly used externally by applying a few drops to the affected area, for instance, a few dabs to the temples or the occipital area for headache.

Internally it can be used prudently for the initial stage of a wind invasion. Put a few drops in an 8 oz (235 ml) glass of water and drink. This can expel the pathogen, reduce swelling and inflammation of the glands, and relieve a sore throat. Avoid contact with mucous membranes.

Po Sum On Oil

Po Sum On is an energetically warm liquid as designated by its deep brown color. Like other warm liniments it invigorates the blood and dispels cold. It is good for wind-cold aches and blood stagnation. Mostly it is applied topically such as on the chest when there is a chest cold. A small dab can be put on a cotton swab and applied locally to the teeth and gums temporarily for the pain of a toothache. Avoid eyes and open wounds. Apply liberally and frequently. This liniment, like *Zheng Gu Shui*, is also flammable.

Wan Hua

Wan Hua is a warm brown liquid also used for blood stagnation. As such, it relieves pain, transforms stagnation, and relaxes sinews and tendons. It is excellent for burns, trauma, and bleeding. As the Chinese instructions so aptly put it, it is good for "stricken, fallen, shocken and twisten conditions and not for the pregnants." Even though it is a liquid, it is used on a burn or a cut. Apply several times per day.

Yunnan Pai Yao

Yunnan Pai Yao is a very powerful powder that primarily has an effect on the blood. Its main ingredient of raw pseudo ginseng, which disperses stagnant blood, stops bleeding, invigorates the blood, and stops pain. It is used for traumatic bleeding such as that induced by trauma, cuts, or other wounds. It can be applied to hot skin infections, skin ulcerations, and insect bites. Internally with proper differentiation it can be taken in its capsulated form for ulcers, sore throat, and menstrual cramps. For serious life-threatening wounds with collapse of *yang* administer the little red pill found at the top of the bottle, which has the function of restoring the *yang*.

Bruise and Pain Plaster

Various plasters for bruises have an analgesic function that promotes the circulation of blood, stimulates healing, stops pain, and is cooling. They are used for bruises, fractures, sprains, neuralgia, arthritis, rheumatism, muscle tenderness, muscle strain, and musculoskeletal pain due to wind.

Apply to clean, dry, hair-free skin and retain for a few days. Do not apply to the lower abdomen or low back during pregnancy. Do not use on children under the age of 2. Avoid contact with the eyes. Do not apply to wounds or broken skin and do not affix too tightly. The plaster can get wet in a bath or shower.

Spray Moxa

Spray moxa is a new form of moxa delivery that comes in a non-aerosol spray. It penetrates through the skin and muscle to the channel level. Like other forms of moxa, it moves *qi* and blood and tonifies the *yang*. It is used for joint pain, muscle strain, swellings, and fractures.

Spray the product on the affected area. Note that it feels cold on application so prepare the patient by letting them know this in advance. Because the moxa needs heat to activate it, position the TDP lamp over the area and keep on for about 10 minutes (see Chapter 20 on the TDP lamp and how to use safely and appropriately). You can also apply *Zheng Gu Shui*, a hot liniment, first and then follow with the spray moxa. *Zheng Gu Shui* will heat up the spray moxa as well as assist in its penetration. Do not use during pregnancy.

Ching Wan Hung

Ching Wan Hung is a Chinese ointment that is known as the burn ointment. It promotes circulation of *qi* and blood, cools heat, stops pain immediately, promotes tissue growth, reduces swelling and blistering, prevents infection, deputrifies and acts as a bactericide. It can be used for skin diseases, bedsores, hemorrhoids, sunburn, heat rash, large area deep burns and scalds caused by boiling water, oil, molten steel, fire, steam, or radioactive or chemical substances. It is very useful for the burns received by patients undergoing radiation treatment. Re-apply daily and cover the dressing with a bandage.

Note: Most of these products will stain clothes. The stain can be removed with rubbing alcohol or better yet have the patient wear old clothing when using the liniments. With all products, avoid the eyes and mucous membranes. Except where indicated avoid open wounds. Discontinue if allergic skin reactions or irritation develops. Some of these products can be taken internally. See discussion above or consult standard herbal texts on how to use in this manner. Keep these and all drugs out of the reach of children. In case of accidental ingestion seek professional assistance or contact a poison control center immediately.

19 An Overview of the Therapeutic Application of Moxibustion

Like *yin* and *yang*, the Chinese characters for acupuncture and moxibustion are inextricably linked together in the image of needles and fire:

针
灸

The Chinese word *zhen jiu* (acupuncture and moxibustion), implies that the two techniques are virtually inseparable. They combine well and are mutually enhancing.[1] *The Prescription Worth a Thousand Gold for Emergencies*[2] states, "The doctor is not a good one if he is not good at both acupuncture and moxibustion" and *Miraculous Pivot*[3] makes the astute differentiation that moxa is suitable to treat all conditions that cannot be cured by acupuncture. *Elementary Medicine*[4] continues by saying, "Moxibustion must be applied if the disease cannot be cured by medicine and acupuncture."

This traditional technique treats the body by way of application of mugwort or *Artemisia Chinensis Vulgaris* to the acupuncture points. The power of moxa with its mild heat, and acrid and bitter properties, lies in its ability to penetrate through the skin and the musculature to the channel level. As an actual material substance, a species of chrysanthemum, most physicians maintain that it is more physical and powerful than needles, and hence better suited to augment the body and especially to move blood stasis. As old as acupuncture itself, it has several clinical functions that are a product of its biochemical properties. Each of these unique roles activates the body's natural healing ability.

■ Functions of Moxibustion

While moxibustion can be used as an independent modality, it is not uncommon to combine acupuncture with moxibustion to enhance its therapeutic effect. Compared with needles, moxa is, relatively speaking, more *yang* in nature. Thus, it has the ability to penetrate to the channel level, promote the circulation of *qi* and blood in the channels, and to move *qi* and blood stasis. Additionally, its *yang* nature facilitates expelling wind, cold, and damp pathogens that can precipitate illness characterized by painful obstruction symptoms called *bi*-syndromes.

Moxa has a special effect on white blood cells, whose job it is to ward off infection. It can activate the function of lymphatic tissue that produces white blood cells such as the bone marrow, spleen, tonsils, lymph nodes, and thymus tissue. It not only stimulates white blood cell production, but also maintains them at a high level in the blood. Furthermore, it can increase the speed with which white blood cells travel to an infected or injured area, and increases their ability to perform their functional roles in the body. These functions have been documented serologically.[5]

In treatment, moxibustion can be used for both tonification of vacuity illness or reduction of excess conditions. French acupuncturist and physician Jean Claude Bossy correctly states that "all *xu zheng* (deficiency syndromes) are associated with lowering of the defense system; thus, therapeutics must reinforce general conditions, *zang* conditions and local conditions. Moxa appears essential in the treatment of *xu zheng*."[6] Moxa is an excellent method to use for the prevention of illness as well as the overt treatment of vacuity syndromes, perhaps the preponderance of a clinician's practice.

Specifically, moxa can tonify *yin* and *yang*, *qi* and blood. Moxa can warm the cold, warm the *yang* and elevate the *yang*. It is the treatment method of choice for syndromes due to external cold, cold arising from *yang* vacuity, and to enhance immunity. The classics actually say that the best method for tonification of *yin* is with moxa because *yin* channels carry fire as well as *jing* fluid. For example, the kidney channel carries *yin*, *qi*, *jing*, and *yang*. The application of moxa on a *yin* channel gives it more fire.[7] In fact, *The Miraculous Pivot*[3] maintains, "Deficiency of both *yin* and *yang* should be treated by moxibustion."

Due to its bitter and acrid properties, moxa can be used to dry cold damp as well as resolve damp heat. Contrary to many clinicians' assumptions, moxa is not contraindicated for damp heat as all internally generated dampness comes from a vacuity of the spleen. In fact, the use of moxa is the "secret" to the successful resolution of many damp heat conditions that create intractable damp heat diseases such as dermatological disorders, leukorrhea and yeast infections to name a few. As a result, it relieves swellings and masses by moving *qi* and blood and drying dampness. Moxa may be used for non-cancerous lymph node swellings or breast lumps, however, do not use on hot swellings or malignancies. For quick reference, the following list summarizes these therapeutic usages:

Physiological Properties of Moxibustion

1. Penetrates to the channel level; promotes the circulation of *qi* and blood; moves *qi* and blood stasis; promotes blood and lymphatic circulation;
2. Raises the white blood cell count and sustains it; increases the speed of white blood cells to the affected area; increases the ability of white blood cells to perform their function;
3. Tonifies vacuity of *qi*, blood, *yin*, and *yang*; warms the cold, warms the *yang*, elevates the *yang*. Can be used preventatively; reduces excess;
4. Dries cold damp and transforms damp heat.

Contraindications, Cautions, and Limitations

In Chinese medicine the two basic contraindications for moxibustion are excess heat, and *yin* vacuity with heat or fire. Excess heat characteristics include fever, inflammation, rapid full pulse; red tongue with yellow coat; red face, loud voice, feelings of heat; red, sore throat; red eyes; thirst for large amounts of cold drinks; dark scanty urine, constipation; and anger, agitation, irritability and restlessness.

A stroke can be precipitated if moxa is used on an excessively hot person because moxa increases body temperature, dilates blood vessels and raises blood pressure, so correct diagnosis as always is critical. Excess heat however, is relatively uncommon. In my clinical experience I would maintain that perhaps less than 5 % of the population has this presentation but it does occur. We all tend to have heat in some places, but overall, from an eight-principle perspective, the diagnosis is not excess heat.

Yin vacuity heat symptoms include five-palm heat, malar flush (afternoon fever), night sweats; red tongue with no coat, and a thin, rapid pulse. Moxa used on *yin* vacuity conditions with heat or fire will further consume the proper *yin* and lead to the dangerous development of fire syndromes and exuberance of *yang*. However, there are cases of *yin* vacuity that do not have heat manifestations.

Yin vacuity can be measured on a continuum. There can be *yin* vacuity, *yin* vacuity with heat, or *yin* vacuity with fire. Symptoms of *yin* vacuity without heat include a thin body, dry skin, throat and mouth; small, frequent thirst; fatigue; thin tongue with cracks, and little to no coat; and thin pulse. Moxa can be used in these cases; however, monitor closely for signs of heat aggravation that usually present as agitation, a sensation of heat, and a red tongue.

Historically, when herbal therapeutics took precedence in China, hot herbs of course were contraindicated for hot conditions. But a faulty equation then developed and carried over into acupuncture that moxa was contraindicated for all heat manifestations. This is true if the patient exhibits signs of excess heat or *yin* vacuity with heat or fire, but there is an interesting variety of heat due to *qi* vacuity. Such manifestations include fatigue, spontaneous sweat, and daytime fever worse with exertion. This heat is not of the excess variety or due to *yin* vacuity but rather the overworking of the weakened body's energy that produces a low-level heat. Moxa is not contraindicated for these cases; in fact, it is the method of choice for this condition, that is, to tonify the *qi*. Indeed, the use of moxa as we have seen, is essential to the treatment of the *xu zheng* (vacuity) syndromes.

There are other cautions and limitations that circumscribe the use of moxibustion. The classics admonish us not to treat infants and children under the age of 7 with moxa because it can induce the inter-transformation or even separation of *yin* and *yang*. This means that the already *yang*-natured child could become too hot, and treatment with moxa could result in death.

Exercise caution with patients who have decreased neurological functioning due to nerve damage, diabetes, age, or those with reduced mental status, as they might not be able to report the temperature sensation to you and serious burns could be induced. Certain drugs such as painkillers and steroids may also inhibit pain perception, so as is customary, a thorough medical history is essential.

My personal preference for acupuncture or moxibustion is not to treat during pregnancy. If you choose to use moxa however, under no circumstances should it be applied to the low back or abdomen of the pregnant women, nor on the standard points forbidden to needle or moxa during pregnancy as they may lead to miscarriage.

In general, moxa should be avoided on the face due to the relative delicacy of the facial skin, and the proximity of the heat, smoke, and flame to the hair, nose and eyes. The smell of the moxa may also be noxious to patients with respiratory disorders and allergies or in certain institutional settings or shared professional offices. Smoke detectors might also be activated with the use of moxa, so consider the sensitivities of your patients, the environment in which you work, and your own proclivities as well.

Moxa is contraindicated if used in the proximity of various nerves and prominent blood vessels such as on ST-9 (*ren ying*) as it is directly on the course of the common carotid artery. Less moxa is generally applied on the chest, in hairy areas that can ignite, and near the heart and the neck. The practitioner should be well aware of such points. If you forget, consult the standard acupuncture textbooks before proceeding with treatment or Table 19.**1** of this chapter.

The customary precautions that apply to acupuncture treatment also apply to moxibustion, such as not to administer to the patient who is overtired or overfed. Additionally, do not use before or after a hot bath, with extreme physical fatigue or emotional distress, if too hungry, after alcohol consumption or drug use, or if the patient is allergic to moxa.

■ Methods of Application

There are two discrete styles of moxa application—direct and indirect moxibustion. Both may be employed as an autonomous modality or to augment needle therapy. Direct moxa makes contiguous contact with the skin; indirect moxibustion does not touch the skin.

Direct moxa may purposely be used to cause scarring. This style is also referred to as open or festering moxibustion. It is believed that the mechanism by which it works is through the continuous stimulation of the acupuncture point created by the burn as it is being healed, as well as the elimination of the pathogen through the suppuration. Scarring moxa is used to treat painful joints due to cold and damp, hard masses, arthritis, and scrofula, or chronic, persistent or life-threatening diseases such as asthma or tuberculosis, and the prevention of stroke. Moxa has germicidal properties so that the risk of infection is theoretically fairly minimal when burned on the skin but it is a painful method and can cause a third-degree burn. If the burn becomes infected, especially in those with weakened immunity, the wound must be treated.

Direct non-scarring moxa is also applied to the skin in the form of moxa cones or thread-size moxa. However, the moxa is removed before it creates a burn. This method of application can be used to treat many conditions such as asthma, chronic diarrhea, impaired digestion and more.

Personally I do not believe direct scarring or even direct non-scarring moxa needs to be done on most patients. The risk of burn or its potential is not proportionate to the therapeutic outcome. I neither do it nor recommend it. Exercise caution

Forbidden Acupuncture Points for Moxa	
General	
Moxa is usually contraindicated or limited in the following areas	1. On the facial skin, which is delicate and can easily burn. The tiger thermie warmer is applicable on some of them 2. Close to the sensory orifices and mucous membranes such as the ears, nose, eyes, and mouth, which are sensitive to heat and smoke, and the genital area 3. Generally contraindicated close to major arteries and veins so they are not damaged, or blood flow increased, or on large tendons, which can contract due to the heat. These are frequently found where large creases are on the body such as the elbow, wrist, etc.
Lung	
LU - 3 (*tian fu*)	No moxa—on course of brachial artery. Also as a Window to the Sky point can cause rebellious *qi*
LU - 5 (*chi ze*)	No moxa—may shorten the biceps brachii tendon
LU - 8 (*jing qu*)	No moxa—on the course of the radial artery. Point is located too superficially
Large intestine	
LI - 1 (*shang yang*)	Generally no moxa—usually the point is bled to clear heat
LI - 4 (*he gu*)	No moxa (or needle) in pregnancy
LI - 13 (*shou wu li*)	No moxa—on course of radial collateral artery and vein and nerve
LI - 19 (*kou he liao*)	No moxa—too close to the eyeball
LI - 20 (*ying xiang*)	No moxa—at ala nasi (wing of the nose)
Stomach	
ST - 1 (*cheng qi*)	No moxa—too close to the eyeball and the ophthalmic artery
ST - 2 (*si bai*)	Usually no moxa due to location too close to the eye
ST - 8 (*tou wei*)	No moxa—brings too much energy to the head
ST - 9 (*ren ying*)	No moxa—precisely on course of carotid artery
ST - 17 (*ru zhong*)	No moxa (or needle)—on the nipple
Spleen	
SP - 6 (*sanyin jiao*)	No moxa (or needle) in pregnancy
Small intestine	
SI - 18 (*quan iao*)	No moxa—too close to the eye

Table 19.**1** Points forbidden for moxa

Forbidden Acupuncture Points for Moxa	
Bladder	
BL-1 (*jing ming*)	No moxa—in the inner canthus
BL-2 (*zan zhu*)	No moxa—too close to the eye
BL-3 (*mei chong*) through BL-10 (*tian zhu*)	No moxa due to location close to the eyes and the occipital artery
BL-16 (*du shu*)	No moxa—may cause back spasm
BL-40 (*wei zhong*)	No moxa—due to effect on local tendons
Triple burner	
TB-19 (*lu xi*)	No moxa—within the hairline above the auricle
TB-23 (*si zhu kong*)	No moxa—too close to the eyeball
Gall bladder	
GB-1 (*tongzi liao*)	No moxa—too close to the eyeball
GB-9 (*tian chong*)	No moxa—within the hairline above the auricle
GB-42 (*di wu hui*)	No moxa—some evidence that vessels may become damaged
Conception vessel	
CV-23 (*lian quan*)	Moxa applicable but not commonly performed on the hyoid bone
Governing vessel	
GV-6 (*ji zhong*)	No moxa—affects the spine
GV-7 (*zhong shu*)	Books say not contraindicated but clinically moxa moves spine
GV-15 (*ya men*)	No moxa—at the base of the medulla
GV-25 (*su liao*)	No moxa—on tip of the nose and the proximity of the nasal mucous membranes
GV-26 (*shui gou*)	No moxa—above the lip, at the philtrum directly below nostrils connected to brain
GV-27 (*dui duan*)	No moxa—above the lip and too close to the mouth and the nose
GV-28 (*yin jiao*)	No moxa—on the frenulum inside mouth
Peter Deadman adds: no moxa to: HT-1 (*ji quan*), 2 (*qing ling*), 3 (*shao hai*) due to brachial artery GB-22 (*yuan ye*), 23 (*zhe jin*)due to breast area GB-33 superior genicular artery and vein GV-4 (*ming men*) males under 40	

Table 19.**1** Points forbidden for moxa (cont.)

even with certain forms of indirect moxibustion, which can still cause serious burns if left unattended and if the size and frequency of the moxa is too much, or if the patient is at risk for burns such as a diabetic patient.

Indirect moxa is the most contemporary, common, and practical moxa modality. There are many tools to use for this style of treatment and they will be discussed later in this chapter, but first we will turn to the concepts of tonification and dispersion with moxibustion in general.

Tonification and Dispersion

Remember that moxa may be used to both tonify and disperse although many practitioners think that it is only for tonification. Just as in needling, in order to accomplish these objectives, different parameters are involved. A complete moxa prescription involves the number, size, density, rate of burning, and the amount of time the moxa is burned, and also the selection of the specific acupuncture points, and the actual moxa modalities selected.

Tonification with moxa provides gentle reinforcement to the patient's vacuity condition. There are several ways to achieve this end. In general, if moxa cones are selected, burn in odd incremental numbers such as three or five. Allow them to burn down slowly and naturally (meaning do not blow on them) for less than 5 minutes until the skin is warm. Fewer cones should be used for thin body areas as well as for older, younger, and weaker constitutional types if used at all and then use cautiously. While a smaller amount of moxa is used in tonification, the moxa should be applied for a longer period of time. If using a warming needle technique, burn the same number of cones on the needle.

If other moxa modalities such as the tiger thermie warmer or mini-thread moxas are utilized, small amounts should be adopted but with greater frequency such as two to three times a week. If an indirect moxa pole is preferred, the point should be gently warmed for 5 minutes by holding the stick far enough away from the body so that the acupuncture point stays warm but not hot. If a sparrow-pecking method is used, slowly heat the point by rotating the stick so that the point is gently warmed in a circular movement from outside to inside as you simultaneously move up and down in the sparrow-pecking manner. Hold the stick 0.5 to 1 in away from the point for about 10 seconds, withdraw for a few seconds, and then repeat for a total of 2 to 5 minutes without creating hot heat.

If vacuity is in the lower part of the body (i. e., prolapse, diarrhea), treat the upper part of the body first (i. e., moxa on GV-20, *bai hui*); if it is in the upper part of the body, treat the lower first (i. e., KI-1, *yong quan*). In general, the *yang* portion of the body is treated first, then the *yin*, that is, the back first, then the front; the top first, then the lower portion, the head and then the abdomen, the extremities, and then the torso.

Dispersion methods are roughly the opposite of tonification procedures. As is true with tonification, dispersion is also relative to the person so the amount of moxa used is correlated with the patient's condition. In general, more moxa such as larger cones are selected for dispersion. More thickly muscled areas require more moxa but it should be administered with less frequency. Use between five to ten cones and let them burn out quickly so that skin becomes red but does not burn. Blowing on the moxa or packing the moxa less compactly in a cone will facilitate a quick burn. Another way of achieving the same result is to burn several moxa cones quickly for about five minutes or blow on the cone and then put another on top of it until the skin gets redder. If a moxa pole is selected, use a quick hot method for 5 minutes by rotating the stick outward from the point. To disperse the heat from the moxa, following its removal, rub the skin vigorously with your hand. Remember that while these are standard Chinese techniques they can still be dangerous to use. Table 19.**2** offers a summary of this material.

Moxa Modalities

Over a dozen moxa modalities that the practitioner may select from are now outlined. For ease of comparison they are also summarized in Table 19.**3** located at the end of this section.

Method	Tonification	Dispersion
1. Amount (number), size of cones to use, and rate of burn	Use less for tonification (three to five cones). Let them burn out naturally for less than 5 minutes until the skin becomes mildly red. Use less for thin bodily areas. Use less for old, and young or weak constitutional types but for a longer amount of time and with greater frequency	Use more for dispersion (five to ten cones). Let them burn down quickly by blowing on them until the skin is red but not burned. Use more for dispersing. Use more for thickly muscled areas
2. Indirect moxa pole	Warm the point gently for 5 minutes, holding far enough away so the point stays warm but not hot. Rotate the pole slowly so the point is warmed gently. Make a circular movement from the outside in towards the point. If using a sparrow-pecking movement, hold the stick 0.5 – 1 in away for about 10 seconds while lifting and thrusting. Withdraw for a few seconds and repeat. Do for 2 to 5 minutes without creating hot heat	Use a quick hot method for 5 minutes. Rotate outward from the point
3. Other modalities	Use small amounts such as with the tiger thermie warmer or moxa thread	Use larger amounts such as with the lion thermie warmer
4. Frequency	Two to three times per week or at least every week	Use less frequently

Table 19.**2** Methods of tonification and dispersion with moxibustion

Moxa Cones

Cones are a common method of administering moxa therapy. They may be used in either a scarring or non-scarring manner. As previously discussed, the scarring method tends to be warranted only for very severe conditions such as life-threatening asthma or to increase longevity. In "Notes on Bian Que's moxibustion"[8] it is said that "When a healthy man often has moxibustion to the points *guan yuan* (CV-4), *qi hai* (CV-6), *ming men* (GV-4) and *zhong wan* (CV-12) he would live a long life, at least one hundred years." Remember, the contraindications for this style of moxa. To reduce the pain associated with a scarring technique, scratch the surrounding skin on the patient as a method to disperse the heat.

Moxa cones may also be used in a non-scarring manner as well. This is achieved by the practitioner quickly removing the cone of moxa, the tiger thermie instrument or other moxa implement from the patient's skin as soon as the patient reports that it is hot. The cone should be removed with tweezers and immediately put into an ashtray. Direct non-scarring moxa confers the therapeutic effects of moxa without the permanent cosmetic results produced by scarring. Cones can also be burned on top of a gauze insulation (see insulations discussed later in this chapter).

To prevent infection following these techniques, if there is a large blister, break it with a sterile needle to allow the liquid to drain out; small blisters will be reabsorbed by the body. Then carefully dress the wound with a burn ointment such as *Ching Wan Hung* or *Wan Hua* and cover with a gauze pad. Change the dressing daily until the burn heals but monitor closely so that it does not become infected. I have seen irreversible acid reflux disease and hypertension caused by Chinese doctors with the overuse of moxa cones, so use judiciously.

Thread Moxa

Thread moxa is a Japanese modality. It comes in at least three sizes—small, medium, and large. It is especially useful in the treatment of *yin* vacuity because it is small and can be applied precisely to a point to confer the healing effects of moxa. Put a small amount of *Ching Wan Hung* or Vaseline on the skin to hold the thread moxa and then position the thread vertically on top of the ointment.

Because the thread is so small it must be ignited with a small incense stick. The flame from a lighter or a match is too large—there is the risk of burning the patient with a larger implement.

Moxa on Needles

On the needle is a primary way in which moxa is used in Chinese medicine. Metal handle needles, not plastic, must be used to burn the moxa. Silver needles work well at conducting the heat but stainless steel is also effective. This method is ideal for directing heat precisely into a particular point such as joints to promote the circulation of *qi* and blood through the channels, to remove external cold, wind, or damp, which can stagnate *qi* and blood flow, and to tonify cold due to *yang* vacuity. Specific instances of this application are to treat wind, cold, damp, and cold damp resulting in *bi*-syndromes, or general weakness, cold, numb limbs, diarrhea, or abdominal distention. Ignite from the bottom of the cone, not the top, to facilitate proper burning.

Apart from moxa on needles, moxa caps, loose impure moxa positioned on top of an ash catcher, or pre-cut (formed) moxa with or without an ash catcher are alternative modalities. An ash catcher can easily be made with a piece of cardboard. Carefully retrieve the ash so that the hot embers do not fall on the patient's skin and cause burns.

The Moxa Burner (or Iron)

This is an interesting style of moxa delivery. Before using the brass burner, first put a piece of cloth (the Chinese recommend red flannel) or several layers of gauze on top of the skin to be treated. The cloth or gauze is used as a method of insulation to protect the patient from being burned. The surface area of the burner allows for a broad area of the body to be treated. In this way it is useful to treat musculoskeletal problems such as spasms and muscular tightness.

Fill the burner with several grams of crude or semi-crude moxa and light with a match. Then, like an iron, move the burner back and forth over the cloth on the affected area. Do not touch the brass burner or allow it to come in contact with unprotected skin—the brass is an efficient conductor of the moxa heat but can cause serious burns to the patient and the practitioner.

The Moxa Box

The moxa box is one of the most ingenious methods of moxa usage, devised for the expansive areas of the back and the abdomen. It is especially effective for the treatment of external cold and *yang* vacuity. The two primary locations for the positioning of the moxa box are on the bare skin of the abdomen from CV-9 (*shui fen*)—CV-4 (*guan yuan*) area and the low back in the BL-23 (*shen shu*) to BL-25 (*da chang shu*) area. Do not place the moxa box on the mid-back or it can cause muscular spasm.

Take a moxa pole and break it into three equal pieces. Remove the outside decorative paper, which is labeled (not the inner wrapper that holds the moxa in a roll). Take two of these pieces and light each end. Place the cover on the box at an angle such that part of the cover is off to allow oxygen into the box. The rate of the burn can be controlled in this manner. A faster burn is achieved with more of the cover askew and a slower one with less. Burn slowly. Do not cover the box completely or the moxa will go out. Also do not use loose moxa in the box—its low density will cause it to ignite and burn too quickly. Over a 10 to 20 minute period check the skin beneath the box about every 5 minutes to see that it is mildly warm and not causing any burn. As with all moxa, exercise extreme caution with patients who have delicate skin such as the elderly, diabetics, or those on pain medication, and patients with neurological deficits or mental impairment who may not be able to report a temperature sensation.

Moxa boxes can cause very serious burns. The practitioner should never let the patient adjust the box or remove the box him/herself. The practitioner should always be in line of sight to monitor the patient's reaction to the moxa box.

The Belly Bowl

The belly bowl is a Korean adaptation analogous to the moxa box. The belly bowl is specifically for using on the navel although clinicians do use it on other areas. It is a small round metal apparatus that has a large single hole or several small holes in which the moxa is placed. The bigger hole is used on the navel and allows for more concentrated heat; more diffuse heat is achieved with the smaller ones. Like the moxa box, monitor the patient carefully when using the belly bowl because it can burn the delicate navel easily. Do not use the belly bowl on navels that are "outies" as they will burn because of their outward configuration.

This modality facilitates tonification with its slow consistent heat, thereby warming the cold and the *yang*. It is especially useful for the treatment of loose stools, undigested food, gas, bloating, menstrual cramps, cold in the uterus, infertility, impotence, cold hands and feet, frequent urination, incontinence, low back pain, and muscle spasm.

Insulations

An insulation is another method of administering moxa. An insulation is a form of protection that both serves to prevent the heat of the moxa from burning as well as to confer the curing benefits of the moxa and the insulated material. Historically, various substances have been used for this effect. They include, but are not limited to, clay, ginger, garlic, leeks, aconite, white mustard seed, miso, wine or water, salt, tangerine peel, tissue, and gauze.

Clay has the medicinal effect of drying due to its astringent properties. A cake of clay can be placed on the area of the body to be treated such as on damp skin suppurations and then a cone of moxa placed over it and ignited. The heat of the moxa will further assist in the drying aspect of the clay. Dermatological conditions such as eczema can be treated in this manner. Adjust the size and frequency of administration to the clinical condition.

Moxa on ginger is a classical method of moxa application to augment *yang* vacuity. The *yang* nature of the moxa with the *yang* characteristics of the ginger (*Recens Zingiberis Officinalis*) is ideal to strengthen the *yang* synergistically. Points that energetically regulate *yang* function such as ST-25 (*tian shu*) as in the case of chronic loose stools, or the navel to directly treat the spleen and kidney *yang* vacuity as manifested through cold hands and feet, loose stools with undigested food, painful menses, constipation, abdominal pain, malabsorption of nutrients, allergic rhinitis, and external cold invasion should be treated with this method.

Cut a piece of raw, fresh ginger root about 0.25 – 0.5 in thick, and perforate it several times with a needle. Position the ginger on an acupuncture point such as CV-4 (*guan yuan*) or CV-6 (*qi hai*) and place a cone of moxa on top of it. Light the moxa and allow it to burn. The heat and resin of the moxa as well as the fresh ginger juice will be deposited on the skin via the holes. Use three to five cones per slice of moxa. If needed, turn the ginger over to assist in the secretion of more resin and juice.

Garlic has antibacterial and antiviral properties that can be utilized along with the use of moxibustion. Therapeutically, it can be used to treat parasites, poisonous insect bites, skin ulcers, boils, and carbuncles. Perforate the garlic with a needle in several places. Then place a piece of wet tissue or paper towel on the area to be treated and the clove of garlic on top of it. Next put a cone of moxa on top of the garlic and light. Garlic can be insulated with miso paste too.

The garlic can be crushed and made into a paste on which to burn the moxa cones. Leeks may be similarly used. A paste of powdered aconite (*fu zi*, Radix Aconiti), the hottest Chinese herb, can be used to warm the *yang* as in the case of a cold ulcer, impotence, and nocturnal emission. White pepper powder mixed with flour can be used in the same manner.

Salt is a common moxa insulation, which is suitable only for the navel to aid the moxa in directly penetrating to the kidney area. It is used for interior cold conditions such as kidney *yang* vacuity, or chronic cold due to weak *ming men* fire. The navel can treat many kidney *yang* vacuity symptoms as well as the lung and spleen because the navel pertains to the spleen according to the *Nan Jing* five-element map, and the spleen, as the figurative mother of lung and the grandmother of kidney, can treat each of them.

Ideally, use unprocessed sea salt that contains trace minerals, or pan-fried salt, which has lower water content. A dual-ply tissue may be used as an insulation to guard against burning the interior of the delicate navel. Simply place the tissue over the navel and then put the salt on it. The weight of the salt will sink to fill the size of the navel. Then place the moxa cone on the salt. Burn as many cones of moxa as deemed necessary. When the treatment is complete, simply lift the tissue to easily remove the salt. Remove the cones with a pair of tweezers. Place the used cones in a cup or ashtray. Be careful not to burn the patient. Because the salt conducts the heat so well remove the cones as soon as the patient perceives heat, as it will continue to heat the point while you are removing the cone. If the salt gets too hot, touch the salt with the tweezers to absorb some of the heat or remove the salt.

This method can cause a painful burn that is difficult to heal because of its location. This type of insulation can be used to treat the lack of will to live, abdominal pain, diarrhea, dysentery, pain around the umbilicus, an imperceptible pulse, excess sweat, cold limbs, allergies, skin and respiratory diseases, and damp heat conditions.

Tangerine peel insulation is useful to release external invasions as in the case of the common cold. In particular, place moxa on GV-14 (*da zhui*), point of greatest *yang* of the body, to mobilize the *yang* to expel cold pathogens.

Moxa Stick-ons

Stick-ons are pre-cut and pre-formed moxa sticks that can be placed on an acupuncture point. They are insulated with cardboard and come mixed with a variety of other ingredients such as ginger, cloves, cinnamon, aloe, miso, and garlic, which make the smoke less acrid and pungent. Moreover, they bestow the benefits of the other ingredients. This moxa method can ensure treatment precision and is convenient for administration at home.

Moxa Poles

Poles are virtually identical to moxa sticks in terms of therapeutic use and are very common methods of indirect moxa administration. They can be used on all points for which moxa is suitable. Make sure to tell the patient to take the exterior paper off before burning if they take them home to use or it could be very dangerous because it will ignite. Moxa sticks are available in smokeless and non-smokeless varieties; the smokeless form is created by densely packing the moxa and mixing it with other ingredients as in the stick-on types. It is very difficult to light so the practitioner should procure a butane lighter for office use.

Tiger Thermie/Lion Thermie Warmers

These warmers are Japanese implements used to deliver the healing benefits of moxibustion. Additionally, the metal tool is used in a dredging or stroking manner to break up obstruction mechanically. The lion thermie warmer is larger than the tiger thermie warmer and thus creates considerably more smoke. I personally prefer the smaller instrument. An additional benefit of the tiger thermie warmer is that the patient can use it for safe and gentle self-administration of moxa. This type of moxa may be carefully used on the face around the sinus areas, and on points that tonify *yin* such as Kidney 6 (*shao hai*). Common regions to use the tiger thermie warmer on are the infraorbital and supraorbital areas to treat sinusitis and rhinitis; around the navel for lung, spleen, and kidney disorders; on the posterior border of the sternocleidomastoid muscle for swollen glands, ear infections, neck problems, and external invasions, and around scars to break up stagnation.[9] Apply for approximately 1.5 minutes to each point or area.

Spray Moxa

Spray moxa is a fascinating and modern moxa innovation. It comes in a non-aerosol dispenser and can easily be sprayed on the areas where moxa is used such as muscular zones, joints, bruises, swellings, and fractures. In order to "activate" the functions of moxa, a heat source needs to be employed. Personally I like to apply the spray moxa to the affected area and then place the TDP lamp over that area of skin for 10–20 minutes. When the TDP lamp is not available (as in home administration), I first put a layer of liniment like *Zheng Gu Shui*, the hottest liniment, on the affected area to penetrate through the skin to the channel and even the bone level, to open to the exterior and heat the body. Then I put a layer of spray moxa over it. In this way the restorative function of the moxa may be tapped. The reverse layering can also be used, however, one disadvantage of the spray moxa is that it tends to feel cold upon application, hence I prefer the former method. Because of this feature, let the patient know in advance how it will feel when you apply it so they are prepared for the cold sensation and do not cramp up.

Loose Moxa

Loose moxa commonly referred to as moxa wool, is of course one of the oldest moxa modalities. It comes in various grades ranging from super-pure,

pure, semi-pure, to crude or impure. The more refined the moxa, the lighter its color, the fluffier it is, the faster it burns and the less smoke it makes. The higher the grade of moxa, the more expensive it is. Crude moxa should be used in moxa burners. Only pure moxa should be selected for direct scarring methods to reduce the chance of infection. The best moxa is 3 to 7 years old and has a pleasant, fresh smell. Moxa cones can range from wheat size to about the size of a kernel of corn. The size one makes is dependent upon the condition of the patient. Texts can be consulted on how to roll moxa cones.

Liquid Moxa

Liquid moxa is also a useful form of moxa. It is especially beneficial for swellings and bruises and has energetics similar to *Zheng Gu Shui* or *Tieh Ta Yao Gin*. It disperses blood and fluid stagnation, invigorates *qi* and blood, stops pain, and relaxes tendons and muscles. It may be applied to bone spurs, muscular aches and pains, bruises, and arthritic conditions. Apply generously with a cotton ball to the affected area and let it dry naturally. Avoid mucous membranes and open wounds. Do not use with massage. Do not bandage or warm up except externally with the TDP lamp. Applying after a hot bath is useful to assist in the penetration of the liquid. Liquid moxa will stain clothes.

Electrical Moxa Apparatuses

These are also a new variety of moxa application. Clinically they may not be as effective as the traditional methods outlined above but the reader is encouraged to try all of these methods and to gain his/her own clinical experience. I have not used them and hence cannot evaluate their effectiveness.

Moxa Candy

This is the latest moxa innovation that I was recently exposed to by my students. Leave it to them. It tastes like green tea. All I can say is—I'll take chocolate! Table 19.**3** summarizes all these methods of applying moxa.

Moxa Modalities	Clinical Differentiation	Contraindications/Cautions
Moxa cones	a. Scarring for life-threatening disorders or longevity; b. Non-scarring—powerful moxa method for all reasons moxa is used	Avoid infection of burns if scarring method is used
Thread moxa	a. For vacuity in general or *yin* in particular; b. For point preciseness	Light with an incense stick to prevent burns
Moxa on needles/moxa caps	a. For joint pain; b. Bi-syndromes; c. *Yang* vacuity or external cold	Avoid ashes falling on patient
Moxa burner	To treat broad areas such as muscular areas	Avoid burns to self and the patient. Do not touch the hot burner
Moxa box	For the abdomen and low back	Do not apply to mid-back, will lead to spasm; caution with elderly, diabetics, patients with neurological or mental impairment and delicate skin
Belly bowl	For the navel or discrete areas	Avoid burns to the delicate navel area

Table 19.**3** Moxa modalities: clinical use and contraindications/cautions

Moxa Modalities	Clinical Differentiation	Contraindications/Cautions
Insulations:		
Clay	Dries damp such as with skin disorders	___
Ginger	To augment the *yang* such as for spleen and kidney *yang* vacuity	___
Garlic/Leeks	Antibacterial; antiviral. For insect bites, parasites and skin disorders	___
Salt	Collapsed kidney *yang*, kidney and spleen *yang* vacuity, lung *qi* vacuity	Avoid burning navel
Tangerine peel	Open to the exterior	___
Tissue or gauze	To insulate salt or the moxa burner	___
Aconite	Warms the kidney *yang*	___
White pepper	To warm the *yang*	___
Moxa stick-ons	a. Point precise; b. Mixture of other therapeutic ingredients; c. Convenient take-home therapy	Light before applying or ignite with an incense stick
Moxa poles/Smokeless moxa	a. Virtually all places; b. Low to no smoke; mixture of other therapeutic ingredients	1. Hard to ignite the smokeless type; 2. Remove burned ash quickly so as not to burn the patient
Tiger thermie/ Lion thermie warmers	a. For the neck, navel, sinus areas; b. For points that treat *yin* vacuity	
Spray moxa	For bruises, fractures, muscular aches and pains, swellings	Goes on cold. Need to activate with a heat source
Loose moxa		
Crude	For moxa burners	Do not cause burns
Semi-crude	For tiger thermie warmers and moxa rolls	Do not cause burns
Pure	For direct scarring or non-scarring method	Minimize risk of infection by dressing burns
Liquid moxa	a. Penetrates to the channel level: moves *qi* and blood, dispels cold, warms *yang* b. For swellings, bruises, muscular aches and pains, disperses blood and fluid stagnation, moves *qi* and blood, stops pain, relaxes tendons and muscles	Avoid mucous membranes and open wounds. Do not use with massage; do not bandage or heat up. Will stain clothes
Electrical moxa apparatuses	No smoke	___
Moxa candy	Take internally	___

Table 19.**3** Moxa modalities: clinical use and contraindications/cautions (cont.)

Important: If any variety of moxa therapy is prescribed for self-administration for treatment at home, be sure to provide the patient with clear written instructions on the type, frequency, and duration of moxibustion, as well as contraindications and instructions on what to do in case of questions or accidental burn or injury.

Moxa Prescriptions

The therapeutic use of moxa for specific clinical conditions is too voluminous to list. There are many possible points to use moxa on based upon their energetics and the functions of moxa. Likewise, Oriental medical theory dictates that we treat what we see and treat the whole person, so it is impossible to predict this. Thus the practitioner is left to his/her diagnostic skills and treatment predilection to devise his/her treatment plans. He/she is also encouraged in particular to read journal articles that present the latest clinical information on the topic. In Table 19.**4** I have listed a repertoire of favorite points that lend themselves to the extraordinary, diverse clinical use of this versatile and powerful herb.

Points	Energetics	Notes
GV-14 (*da zhui*) ST-36 (*zu san li*) LI-4 (*he gu*) TB-5 (*wai guan*) BL-12 (*feng men*) BL-23 (*shen shu*) CV-17 (*shan zhong*) CV-4 (*guan yuan*) GV-4 (*ming men*) BL-43 (*gao huang*)	A repertoire of tonic points to strengthen immunity for immune-deficient patients and to increase white blood cell production	Use a non-scarring method. Moxa BL-12 and GV-14 until the skin feels warm. Use small cones, few moxas, and monitor for heat aggravation, as immune-deficient patients often have *yin* vacuity also. Use mild moxa on CV-17 due to its proximity to the heart (i.e., indirect pole or three moxas)
ST-36 (*zu san li*) CV-4 (*guan yuan*) CV-6 (*qi hai*) GV-4 (*ming men*)	Points to increase longevity	Moxa each every other day for 10 minutes to increase T-lymphocytes. Monitor for heat manifestations
KI-1 (*yong quan*)	To tonify the kidney	Apply with the tiger thermie warmer with pressure
TB-16 (*tian you*) KI-6 (*shao hai*) LI-10 (*qu chi*) GV-14 (*da zhui*)	Known as the tonsillar treatment* strengthens immunity by activating lymphatic tissues	Moxa everyday for 1 to 4 months. Moxa each point 1.5 minutes each with the tiger thermie warmer. Moxa KI-6 two to three times for 2 to 3 seconds
BL-23 (*shen shu*) BL-28 (*pang guan shu*) BL-32 (*ci liao*) CV-3 (*zhong ji*) CV-4 (*guan yuan*)	Chronic cystitis	The moxa box or the belly bowl works well here. Apply daily for 15 to 20 minutes until symptoms resolve

If more than one area of the body is treated, do not heat for more than 20 minutes.
* See References, note 5.

Table 19.**4** Moxa prescriptions

Points	Energetics	Notes
SP-1 (*yin bai*)	Abnormal uterine bleeding	To stop, apply moxa for 20 minutes
LI-15 (*jian yu*)	Shoulder osteoarthritis	Insert the needle and add moxa to the handle. Heat the point three times for 5 minutes
LI-11 (*shou san li*)	Osteoarthritis of the elbow	—
LI-5 (*yang xi*)	Osteoarthritis of the thumb	—
TB-4 (*yang chi*)	Osteoarthritis of the wrist	—
GB-30 (*huan tiao*)	Osteoarthritis of the hip joint	—
BL-39 (*wei yang*), extra point *xian*	Osteoarthritis of the knee	—
ST-41 (*jie xi*) ST-42 (*chong yang*)	Osteoarthritis of the ankle	—
GV-14 (*da zhui*) or GV-13 (*yu men*) BL-11 (*da shu*)	Osteoarthritis of the neck	—
ST-7 (*xia guan*)	Osteoarthritis of the jaw	—

Table 19.**4** Moxa prescriptions (cont.)

References

1. Van Alphen J, editor. *Oriental Medicine, an Illustrated Guide to the Asian Arts of Healing*. Boston, MA: Shambhala Publications; 1995:189.
2. Cheng X. The prescription worth a thousand gold for emergencies. In: Cheng X, chief editor. *Chinese Acupuncture and Moxibustion*. Beijing: China Foreign Language Press; 1999:361.
3. Cheng X. Miraculous pivot. In: Cheng X, chief editor. *Chinese Acupuncture and Moxibustion*. Beijing: China Foreign Language Press; 1999:361.
4. Cheng X. Elementary medicine. In: Cheng X, chief editor. *Chinese Acupuncture and Moxibustion*. Beijing: China Foreign Language Press; 1999:361.
5. Nagano K. Immune enhancement through acupuncture and moxibustion: specific treatment for allergic disorders, mild infectious disease and secondary infections. *Amer J Acu*. 1991;19(4):329–338.
6. Bossy J. Immune system, defense mechanisms and acupuncture: fundamental and practical aspects. *Amer J Acu*. 1990;18(3):219.
7. Dzung TV. The curious meridians. *Amer J Acu*. 1989;17(1):45–56.
8. Cheng X. Notes on Bian Que's moxibustion. In: Cheng, X, chief editor. *Chinese Acupuncture and Moxibustion*. Beijing: China Foreign Language Press; 1999:363.
9. Gardner-Abbate S. *The Art of Palpatory Diagnosis in Oriental Medicine*. London: Churchill Livingstone, 2001.

20 The Mineral Infrared Therapy Device

The TDP lamp or mineral infrared therapy device is an instrument originating from China that has won numerous international awards for the treatment of diverse medical conditions. An integral part of the lamp, which when heated emits electromagnetic waves in the infrared range, stimulates the body to heal by influencing the body's trace minerals. Cells below the skin level then absorb these trace elements.

In an acupuncturist's repertoire of tools, the TDP lamp is one of the most expensive tools but is still very affordable, ranging from $175 to $350 depending upon whether a desk lamp model or a freestanding unit is used. After 1500 hours of use, the mineral plate loses its emission ability and needs to be replaced.

The TDP lamp is useful for the treatment of both musculoskeletal and internal disorders. Its various properties are listed below as are the conditions it can treat.

Functions of the Mineral Infrared Therapy Device

- accelerates the decomposition of unstable or dead cells;
- balances the nervous system;
- decreases inflammation and edema;
- improves microcirculation;
- increases enzyme activity;
- eases pain;
- promotes cell growth;
- promotes metabolism.

Illnesses Well-treated with the Mineral Infrared Therapy Device

- acute adult diarrhea;
- angina;
- back pain, lumbago;
- Bell's palsy;
- burns, frostbite, skin ulcers;
- chronic bronchitis;
- dysmenorrhea;
- earache;
- infantile diarrhea;
- insomnia;
- irregular menstruation;
- localized areas of the body;
- mumps;
- muscular pain;
- pelvic inflammation;
- periodontitis;
- prostatitis;
- rheumatic arthritis;
- sinusitis;
- skin disorders such as eczema, tinea, bedsores, herpes and alopecia;
- soft tissue injury.

To use the infrared lamp, pre-heat it before use for about 5 to 10 minutes. When using the lamp, position it 12 to 18 in from the site to be treated. Manufacturer's instructions recommend heating the treatment area for 20 to 30 minutes, however, I am more cautious with its use yet still obtain the same good clinical results. I recommend heating the area for 10 minutes and monitoring the heat by touching the patient's skin after 5 minutes and then continue treatment. If needed the lamp can be used one to two times a week.

There are cautions and contraindications that need to be noted in the use of the lamp and they are listed below:

1. If used incorrectly the lamp may cause serious burns. Never touch the lamp to see that it is heating up.
2. Do not use on patients who are insensitive to pain due to decreased neurological functioning such as diabetics, AIDS patients, those with peripheral neuropathy, those who are on pain medications or others who cannot report a temperature sensation to you.
3. Do not leave the lamp unattended for patients who are incapacitated such as those who are paralyzed or in wheelchairs.
4. Monitor skin temperature to assure the temperature is warming not burning.

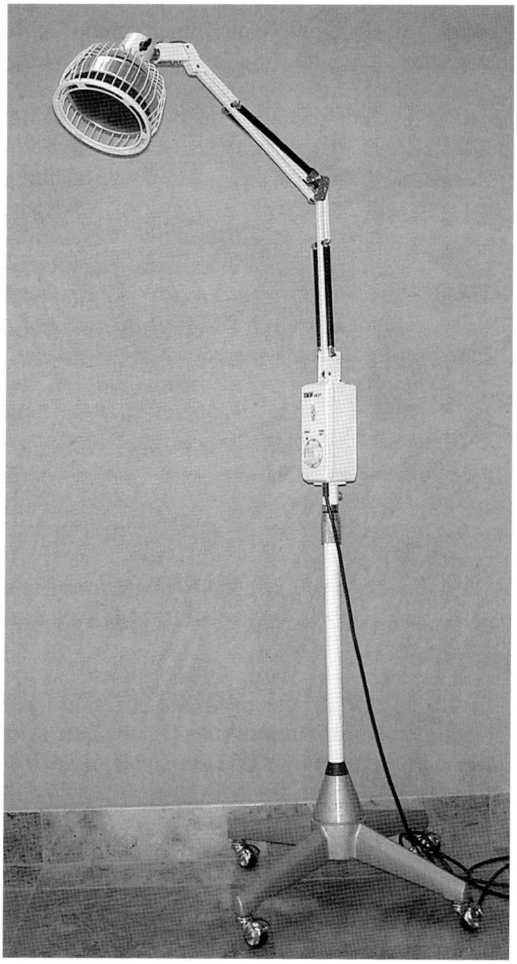

Fig. 20.**1** The TDP lamp.

5. Do not use on patients with high fever, serious arteriosclerosis, a tendency to bleed, or on the head of patients with hypertension.
6. Protect the eyes when used for facial treatment.
7. Do not let children operate or have access to the heated lamp.

The mineral infrared therapy device is an excellent substitute for moxibustion if the patient or practitioner do not like to use moxa for any reason. However, all the contraindications that apply to moxa hold true here as well (see Chapter 19 on moxibustion). Figure 20.**1** depicts the TDP lamp. See the Supplier section at the end of the book on where the TDP lamp may be purchased.

21 Practical Threading Therapy

Through-and-through collective loci treatment, commonly known as threading, is a simple procedure in which two or more acupuncture points are joined together with one needle, or whereby a point that has a relatively large size can be stimulated through the angle of insertion of the needle. Depending upon the points to be threaded, they are either needled subcutaneously (i. e., horizontally along the skin), or perpendicularly through the point.

Threading is a part of treatment options practiced by doctors in China. The Chinese translation of the technique is "one needle for two points." Originally, the purpose of many Chinese threading techniques was to treat difficult and chronic conditions by connecting effective groupings of nearby points together to stimulate the affected area or energetics of those points. The number of points this procedure can be applied to is theoretically broad but in the average Western clinical practice somewhat small.

The most comprehensive exposure that I have had to this method of treatment is in the now out-of-print book, *Through-and-through Collective Loci Acupuncture*[1] and the reader is encouraged to consult that or other books on threading if this method is of interest. The emphasis in this chapter is on subcutaneous needle insertion of the points that I frequently thread in clinical practice. My choice of points to thread, although not extensive, is not complicated or difficult to execute, but can be quite useful when these clinical situations are encountered. The purpose of my adapted techniques is:

- to reduce the number of needles required for treatment, which can be a desirable treatment strategy for many reasons such as treating needle-sensitive patients, or needing to limit the number of needles in the treatment in consideration of the other points chosen to needle;
- as a subcutaneous technique to reduce the needle stimulus and make treatment easier for the patient to tolerate;
- to accomplish efficiently the therapeutic aim of treatment.

The points selected are safe to use and pose virtually no hazard to needle. However, with this unique style of needling there are some general precautions that should be followed:

- Inform the patient that you will be connecting nearby points by needling very shallowly. This technique, at least with the points selected here, is painless. As a reference point, let the patient know that no *de qi* is elicited, perhaps in contrast to other treatments they may have received in the past, so that they can understand the needling sensation.
- Instruct the patient not to move the parts of the body that are needled. As always position the patient in a comfortable position to avoid bending or breaking the needle.
- Be knowledgeable of regional anatomy for the purposes of needling.
- Always needle slowly to control the angle and depth of insertion. Withdraw the needle or change the direction of the needle if you encounter any resistance.
- After withdrawal of the needle, press the treated area with a clean cotton ball to prevent any bruising.

Common Points to Thread

LI-20 (*Yin Xiang*) to *Bi Tong* (Extra Point)

Application

LI-20 can be threaded to the extra point *bi tong* for the treatment of sinusitis and allergic rhinitis with concomitant symptoms of nasal congestion or runny nose, facial itchiness, and swelling.

Location

LI-20—in the nasolabial groove, at the level of the midpoint of the ala nasi. *Bi tong*—at the end of the nasolabial groove, superior to LI-20.

Method

With a #1 gauge 30 mm Seirin needle, thread the points by puncturing LI-20 subcutaneously towards *bi tong*. Connect the points transversely. Needle slowly, shallowly, and with control as you approach *bi tong* in the infraorbital area, threading the needle about 0.5 to 0.75 in. Do not obtain *qi* nor tonify nor disperse, just connect the points.

If the patient has a deep groove or wrinkle in this area, an intradermal needle can be chosen in place of needles. Select several 6 mm Seirin intradermal needles and position them back to back from LI-20 to *bi tong*. Use splinter tweezers or forceps to insert the needles. Have the patient close their eyes or even better, cover their eyes with a small pillow or cotton balls in case you lose control of the minute needles that might accidentally fly towards the patient's eyes.

In either case of using intradermal needles or a regular acupuncture needle, treat bilaterally. Retain the needles for 10 minutes. Remove the intradermal needle with tweezers or forceps. Pull out all of the needles slowly and press the skin with a clean cotton ball to close the holes to reduce infection and prevent bruising.

KI-6 (*Zhao Hai*)—Alternative Location

Application

Use KI-6 for all of the common indications of KI-6 as the point of greatest *yin* of the body. It is indicated for laryngitis, pharyngitis, chronic sore throat, night sweats, hot flushes, diabetes, amenorrhea, declining vision in the aged, insomnia, neurasthenia, itching, and other symptoms of kidney vacuity, especially kidney *yin* vacuity.

Location

The alternative Chinese location of KI-6 (*zhao hai*), commonly referred to as the Japanese location, is the point to be threaded. It is found 1 *cun* below the medial malleolus at the junction of the red and the white skin (see Fig. 3.**1a**, and **b** in Chapter 3).

Method

Puncture the point with a #1 g 30 mm Seirin needle 0.1 to 0.3 *cun* posteriorly and subcutaneously towards the heel. Do not obtain *qi*. The angle of insertion is considered a tonification technique as the point is needled in the direction of the meridian. Treat bilaterally. Retain the needle for 10 minutes.

If preferred, one 3 mm intradermal needle may be inserted during treatment in place of the regular acupuncture needle. Insert and withdraw in the same manner as described under the discussion of LI-20.

BL-2 (*Zhan Zu*) to *Yu Yao* (Extra Point)

Application

Pain in the supraorbital region, redness, swelling and pain of the eyes, sinus or frontal headache, blurry vision, sinusitis, acute conjunctivitis, and allergy symptoms.

Location

BL-2—on the medial extremity of the eyebrow, in the supraorbital notch. *Yu yao*—in the middle of the eyebrow, when one is looking straight ahead, the point is directly above the pupil.

Method

Insert a #1 g 30 mm needle and thread shallowly 0.1 to 0.2 in through BL-2 to *yu yao*. Do not obtain *qi* nor tonify nor disperse. Treat bilaterally. Retain the needle for 10 minutes.

KI-27 (*Shu Fu*) to ST-13 (*Que Pen*)

Application

This is an interesting treatment technique to activate the functions of these two powerful points. I use them frequently in this way to strengthen immunity and treat prolapses (viewed as weak connective tissue due to weakened immunity). They can be selected to treat cough, asthma, chest pain, bronchitis, and prolapses.

Location

KI-27—in the depression on the lower border of the clavicle, 2 *cun* lateral to the *ren* channel. ST-13—at the lower border of the middle of the clavicle on the mammillary line, 4 *cun* lateral to the *ren* channel.

Method

With a #1 g 40 mm Seirin needle, puncture the skin at KI-27 and slowly thread the needle subcutaneously and laterally towards ST-13. The needle will stimulate the ST-13 area. Keep the needle horizontally in the skin tissue due to the proximity of the lungs. Do not obtain *qi* or tonify or disperse. Simply connect the points as you thread the needle about an inch away from KI-27. Needle towards the lateral aspect of the body. Retain the needle 10 minutes. Due to its length, withdraw the needle slowly.

HT-7 (*Shen Men*)—Alternative Location

Application

For anxiety, nervousness, constipation due to nervousness, palpitations, cardiac pain, irritability, mental disorders, hysteria, insomnia, pain in the hypochondriac region, dream disturbed sleep, and depression.

Location

HT-7 alternative (Japanese) location—at the transverse crease of the wrist on the ulnar side of the tendon of the muscle flexor carpi ulnaris in the articular regions of the pisiform and the ulnar bones

Method

Insert a #1 g 30 mm Seirin needle 0.2 to 0.3 in under the tendon towards the standard Heart 7 location. This treatment may be performed bilaterally or just on the left side as heart energetics are more left-sided or if the physical problem is also left-sided. Do not obtain *qi* or tonify or disperse. This is a useful technique to use on patients who have arthritic deformities in the wrist area, thus making the standard Heart 7 hard to needle. Retain the needle for 10 to 20 minutes.

PC-6 (*Nei Guan*) to TB-5 (*Wai Guan*)

Application

For local problems such as contracture of the wrist, arm, elbow, and fingers. Stimulates upper burner function.

Location

Standard Chinese locations for both points. PC-6 can be found 2 *cun* above the transverse crease of the wrist between the tendons of the muscle palmaris longus and the muscle flexor carpi radialis. TB-5 is located 2 *cun* above the transverse crease of the wrist between the ulnar and carpal bones.

Method

Insert a #1 g 30 or 40 mm needle perpendicularly 0.8 to 1.2 in from TB-5 to PC-6. This is a deep insertion. Do not obtain *qi* or tonify or disperse. Instruct the patient not to move his/her hands because movement with the needle in this deep can cause pain. It is also possible for the needle to bend or break. The point may be treated unilaterally or bilaterally. Retain for five to ten minutes.

LU-7 (*Lie Que*)

Application

To use Lung 7 as a longitudinal *luo* point, that is, to direct the stimulus to the lung organ to treat problems of the lung organ or the proximal portion of the lung.

Location

Standard Chinese location, 1.5 *cun* above the transverse crease of the wrist in the depression on the styloid process of the radius.

Method

Insert a #1 or #3 g needle transversely and proximally, that is, up the arm. Obtain *qi* through lifting and thrusting in a transverse manner. When *qi* is obtained, tonify or disperse the needle depending upon the aim of treatment. The stimulus should be directed up the arm.

Lan Wei (Extra Point)

Application

Paralysis, motor impairment of the lower extremities, appendicitis.

Location

2 *cun* below ST-36 (*zu san li*).

Method

Puncture the point subcutaneously with a #3 or #5 g 2 to 3 in needle from *lan wei* downward. Insert slowly and thread the needle through the skin. With a horizontal lift and thrust method, subcutaneously obtain a strong stimulus down the leg to treat the aforementioned conditions, which require strong stimulation.

ST-38 (*Tia Kou*) to BL-57 (*Cheng Shan*)

Application

For shoulder stiffness and motor impairment of the shoulder.

Location

Standard Chinese locations for both points. ST-38: 8 *cun* below ST-35 (*du bi*), 2 *cun* below ST-37 (*shang ju xu*) midway between ST-35 and ST-41 (*jie xi*). BL-57—directly below the belly of the muscle gastrocnemius, on the line connecting BL-40 (*wei zhong*) and tendo calcaneus, about 8 *cun* below BL-40.

Method

Puncture ST-38 perpendicularly on the same side of the leg as the side of the affected shoulder problem. Then without looking for *qi*, insert the needle through the point in the direction of BL-57. Use a 3 in #3 or 5 g needle. When the required depth has been achieved, about 2 in into the leg, lift and thrust the needle slowly as you are in the thick musculature. At the same time have the patient lift and mobilize the shoulder. Lift and thrust the needle during the movement of the arm and then withdraw the needle.

The points and methods presented here are not only easy to do, and can augment your treatment style and options, but most importantly may offer gentle, effective medical care to your patients.

Reference

1. Chang D, Yeung CC, Chung CY. *Through-and-through Collective Loci Acupuncture.* Kowloon, Hong Kong: Medical Interflow Publishing House; 1976.

IV Specialized Use of Points

22 Multiple Uses of Auricular Points

As the first organ to develop to its full size and become fully functional approximately 18 weeks after conception, the ear is also the first sense organ to begin working as early as the eighth week in utero. It is an extraordinary sensory organ that not only connects us with the world and each other through the power of hearing, but also serves as a unique and complete microsystem for the diagnosis, prevention and treatment of virtually every human illness.

Physiologically, the ear is a powerful nexus of energy through which all of the 12 main channels either directly or indirectly intersect with the potent eight extraordinary vessels. This accessible energy is encapsulated in hundreds of auricular acupuncture points that make possible the utilization of the ear as an important method of treatment by clinicians. Auricular acupuncture is easy to learn and master, and when accurate point selection and needle technique are applied to the correct diagnosis, it yields dramatic, immediate, and long-lasting results with a high rate of clinical efficacy.

Assuming the clinician knows how to diagnose correctly and differentiate an illness as well as how to locate precisely and select auricular acupuncture points for a prescription, it is interesting to see how versatile the ear acupuncture points are for numerous and unrelated medical conditions due to their multiple, broad-based energetics that are the hallmark of Oriental medicine.

While a general rule of Oriental medicine is to "treat what you see" so that the unique energetic configuration of the individual is responded to, there are still what we might call core ear acupuncture points that the practitioner can frequently use so that the essential features of an illness are addressed. My recommendation is not that practitioners memorize any prescription but rather that they try to discern how each point contributes to the formula. By doing so, they will test their understanding of the etiology, pathogenesis, and signs and symptoms of a disease, and thus be able to select these points effortlessly when such an illness is encountered without the need to even reference the point energetics.

This chapter provides the reader with a comprehensive list of clinically effective formulas for the treatment of 26 common diseases. This information is offered in Table 22.**1** in alphabetized chart form that makes it easy to access and study as well as to visualize the multiple functions of the same points. Certainly the practitioner should not apply these points to treatment without understanding the person's medical history and the specific differentiation of illnesses, which may have several patterns. Correct location of the ear points of course, is essential to the treatment and the reader is encouraged to consult standards in the field or my last book, *Chinese Auricular Acupuncture.*[1] The salient energetics of the core acupuncture points are listed below so that the reader can appreciate their role in the auricular prescription. Finally, in Table 22.**2**, treatment modality options are outlined for the practitioner.

■ Point Energetics

Shen Men

Shen men is the foremost point in the treatment of virtually every disease. Analogous to body *shen men* (Heart 7), ear *shen men's* functions largely pertain to the heart. Like body *shen men*, the earth point and thus the sedation point of the heart channel, ears—*shen men* adds "dampness" to the body. By virtue of this physiological function, it grounds the patient, and calms the spirit, thus putting the patient into a state of receptivity for treatment. It should be the first point treated in any ear acupuncture prescription because of these energetics.

The only contraindications for *shen men* are when there is already excess phlegm or dampness that would compromise the heart and lungs as in the case of COPD (coronary obstructive pulmonary disease) or asthma or bronchitis characterized by excess phlegm. It is not contraindicated in other

Illnesses	Points									
	Shen men	Brain	Sympathetic	Adrenal	Endocrine	Kidney	Liver	Heart	Spleen	Other Points Specified
Anxiety	✓	✓	✓	✓		✓		✓		Diaphragm
Asthma	✓	✓	✓	✓	✓	✓	✓			
Carpal tunnel syndrome	✓	✓	✓	✓		✓	✓	✓		Fingers, Wrist
Cholecystitis	✓	✓	✓							Gall Bladder, Stomach, Diaphragm
Chronic fatigue	✓			✓		✓	✓		✓	Lung
Coronary artery disease	✓	✓	✓			✓		✓		
Diarrhea	✓					✓	✓		✓	Large Intestine, Stomach, Triple Burner
Eczema	✓	✓	✓	✓			✓	✓		Lung
Facial paralysis	✓	✓		✓			✓		✓	Cheek, Diaphragm, Jaw, Triple Burner, Brainstem
Fibromyalgia	✓	✓	✓				✓	✓	✓	Triple Burner, Diaphragm, Relax Muscle
Herpes zoster	✓						✓			Lung, Diaphragm, Local Area
Insomnia	✓	✓				✓	✓	✓	✓	
Irritable bowel syndrome	✓		✓				✓			Large Intestine
Menopause	✓	✓		✓	✓	✓	✓	✓	✓	Ovary
Migraines	✓	✓	✓				✓			Diaphragm, Ear apex
Multiple sclerosis	✓	✓	✓			✓	✓			
Myopia	✓	✓				✓	✓	✓	✓	Eye, Eye 1, Eye 2, Stomach

Table 22.**1** Core acupuncture points for the treatment of common disorders

Illnesses	Points									
	Shen men	Brain	Sym-pa-thetic	Adre-nal	Endo-crine	Kid-ney	Liver	Heart	Spleen	Other Points Specified
Neurodermatitis (chronic lichen simplex)	✓						✓	✓		Lung, Local Area involved
Otitis media	✓			✓		✓	✓		✓	Inner Ear, Mouth
Post-partum depression	✓	✓			✓	✓	✓	✓		Diaphragm
Post-traumatic stress disorder	✓	✓	✓	✓		✓	✓	✓		
Rheumatoid arthritis	✓	✓	✓			✓	✓		✓	
Sciatica	✓		✓				✓			Sciatic
Temporoman-dibular joint disorders	✓	✓	✓				✓		✓	Jaw, Channel involved (i.e., Stomach etc.)
Tinnitus	✓	✓		✓		✓	✓			Diaphragm
Torticollis	✓	✓					✓			Cervical Vertebrae, Dia-phragm, Neck

Table 22.**1** Core acupuncture points for the treatment of common disorders (cont.)

damp disorders such as leukorrhea, eczema, or obesity.

The heart is the supreme commander and governs the blood. Thus all blood disorders of vacuity, stagnation, extravasation, or rebelliousness can be treated with *shen men*. The *Huang Di Nei Jing* reminds us, "When the heart is serene, all pain is negligible" and this function is largely related to the heart's role in blood regulation as well as the strong relationship of the heart to the mind and the spirit. Indeed, *shen men* proves to be a primary point in the treatment of pain.

Because of its internal pathway of "the eye system," the heart also has a strong connection to the eye and can benefit many opthalmological disorders.

Brain

In my opinion, the brain is the second most important auricular point and should be used in almost every ear prescription. The brain controls everything—all bodily systems and parts—and thus it controls pain perception, movement, and the proper functioning of all the organs.

Sympathetic

Sympathetic is another major auricular point, instrumental in balancing the two branches of the autonomic nervous system: the sympathetic and parasympathetic branches. It promotes dilation of blood vessels, which aids in the relief of pain.

Adrenal

Adrenal point strengthens the function of the kidney particularly by controlling adrenal hormones involved in stress reactions. It reduces pain and quells anti-inflammatory responses.

Endocrine

Endocrine, sometimes referred to as the internal secretion point, regulates all the endocrine glands needed for homeostasis of the internal bodily environment. It is useful in all endocrine, i. e., hormonal disorders.

Kidney

Kidney is the organ that encapsulates the person's genetic inheritance (constitution) as well as the state of one's current health. It is useful in all chronic problems. The kidney is the root of the *qi*. It anchors and secures it thus keeping the person healthy and balanced physically and psychologically. Kidney governs all the developmental life phases from conception through puberty and adulthood, to menopause and aging. The kidney governs the anatomical and physiological domains of the back, the knees, the lower burner, the blood, hearing, and the head hair.

Liver

Liver is the organ responsible for the free flow of *qi* in the body, thus it can move stagnation anywhere in the body. The liver, like the heart and kidney, has a close relationship to the blood. While the heart dominates the blood and the kidney aids in its production, the liver stores the blood, releasing it in the daytime and during menstruation and storing it at night.

The liver dominates the tendons and the muscles. The Chinese character for tendon includes the nerves, tendons, and ligaments. Hence, the liver controls any disorder of these structures. The eyes are the external manifestation of the liver and so the liver point is indicated in treatment of eye disorders.

Heart

Many of the functions detailed under *shen men* are also applicable for the heart, but the heart point directly relates to the heart organ/channel complex in Chinese medicine along with all of its voluminous Western usages. The heart point is synergistically reinforced when used with *shen men* but targets the treatment as related to the heart itself.

Spleen

Spleen, like all the organ points, has numerous physiological functions. It dominates the muscles, making it involved in all muscular movement and health. When the spleen is not functioning properly it is involved in the production of damp. The spleen is responsible for a healthy mind and a balanced spirit. As part of the Oriental digestive system, it is the primary organ involved in digestion and assimilation of nutrients.

Supplementary Points

1. Diaphragm is an extremely powerful point. It assists in respiration and in moving the *qi* of the liver. The diaphragm, through its connection with the liver, moves the blood when stagnant. It also can make an inactive auricle reactive, thus it is a good point to use for this reason also.
2. Fingers are an area for all finger disorders.
3. Wrist is a local point for all wrist disorders.
4. Gall bladder pertains to the organ of the gall bladder that regulates the release of bile to the small intestine for digestive purposes. It treats all gall bladder disorders.
5. Stomach pertains to the stomach organ/channel complex. It is vital to the initial breakdown of food.
6. Lung points also have a *zang fu* connection. They are used for all respiratory problems. The lung points contribute to energy level, as the lungs are the master of the *qi*. They are also very applicable in skin problems and the healing of mucous membranes because the lung dominates the skin and the mucous membranes.
7. Large intestine is a local point for all large intestine problems.

8. Triple burner regulates the three burners, their functions and inter-relationships.
9. Cheek is a local point for cheek disorders.
10. Jaw is a local point for jaw disorders.
11. Brainstem is a local point for all functions of the brainstem. Brainstem treats shock and neuro-vegetative disorders.
12. Relax muscle is a specialized point within the liver area. It is a powerful point in pain relief because of this function.
13. Ovary is a local point for problems of the ovaries such as menopause, infertility, ovulatory problems, and more.
14. Ear apex treats liver *yang* rising symptoms such as hypertension and conjunctivitis.
15. Eye is a main local point for all eye disorders.
16. Eye 1 is a clinically effective point for eye problems.
17. Eye 2 is a clinically effective point for eye problems.
18. Inner ear is a local point for inner ear disorders.
19. Mouth point can be used as a local point for mouth diseases including stuttering, aphasia, dysphasia, oral ulcerations and others. The mouth point is also called the anti-fatigue point. One reason is that it is located close to the external auditory meatus, which is a very tender and delicate area and elicits a strong stimulus upon treatment. Secondly, the mouth point when stimulated in a tonifying manner, promotes eating, which gives one the energy derived from food, hence it combats fatigue.
20. Sciatic can be used for treatment of the sciatic nerve.
21. Cervical vertebrae are local points for disorders of the cervical vertebrae.
22. Neck is a local point for neck disorders.

■ Techniques

The practitioner has numerous auricular techniques to choose from depending upon his/her mode of preference, styles he/she may have been taught, or patient compliance. Table 22.**2**, excerpted from *Chinese Auricular Acupuncture*[1] and presented below, summarizes these techniques. Please refer to my text or other ear acupuncture manuals for more detailed information on these modalities and their contraindications.

Modalities	Conditions
Massage	Massage can be applied by the therapist or the patient after the patient is instructed on where and how to massage the ear. Mark the spot to be massaged with a pellet or sterile marking pen
Needles	Needling is the most common auricular therapeutic modality. Needles can be inserted into any point. Insert—get *qi*—then tonify or disperse. Heat is the most desired sign of *qi* arrival. Note: I tend not to needle the heart or brain points because of their strong stimulus. For these points, I substitute pellets. However, it is not contraindicated to needle them
Ear seeds and herbal plasters	Semen vaccaria seeds provide a good stimulus due to their size and density. However, if they are not sterile they can increase the risk of infection. Herbal deposits on the seeds can impart herbal therapeutic benefits
Ear pellets—gold, silver, or other metals	Pellets are a good-size modality for auricular treatment. They provide a perfect stimulus and have the added benefit of being sterile. Additionally, pellets are available in various metals. Therefore, pellets can also be used for their metallurgic properties
Ear tacks	Tacks come in various sizes—extra small, small, medium, and large. The bigger the tack, the stronger the stimulus, so consider patient tolerance when choosing the tack size. There is a higher risk of infection with ear tacks if patients do not have the tacks removed at the proper time

Table 22.**2** Auricular modalities

Modalities	Conditions
Intradermal needles	Intradermal needles are used for areas such as the fingers or vertebral areas. Do not use in depressions in the ear such as the scaphoid fossa. The intradermal needle will not go into a depression easily and may break. Intradermal needles need to be placed on points on a ridge or flat area. Intradermals are available in various lengths. Select the appropriate length based upon the size of the point to be treated
Magnets	Magnets need to be removed at bedtime or if the stimulus becomes too strong for the patient. They are reusable on the same patient. Magnets do not pierce the skin, thus the risk of infection is reduced
Electroacupuncture	Electricity is good for anaesthetizing a point due to the electrical machine's ability to achieve high frequencies that stimulate the point. Do not clean the ear with alcohol before using the point detector for diagnosis, as this will change the ear pathology and the electrical resistance of the ear
Bleeding	Bleeding is used to reduce heat/fire, subdue *yang*, stimulate *qi* and blood, or to move stagnant *qi* and blood
Moxibustion	Moxa use is limited but specific to treat earache or the common cold and other conditions. It can be applied indirectly over the point or with an incense-size moxa stick
Incisions/sutures	Incisions/sutures are a technique that is typically not employed in the Western countries because an incision is considered a surgical technique. An incision provides a constant stimulus to the point. Chances of infection are increased using incisions
Injections	Injections can be applied to the point with a hypodermic needle. Common injections include saline, vitamin B12, certain Chinese herbal formulations, lidocaine, procaine, and placenta. This procedure is slightly painful due to the small size of the point, the size of the hypodermic needle and the nature of the substance injected
Laser	Laser therapy is one of the newest modalities. It is painless and infection is not an issue. Ease of administration also makes it a good choice in treatment
Staples	Like incisions and sutures this is an old technique used to stimulate points. Seeds or pellets are commonly used now in the place of staples
Plum blossom needling	This modality may be applied to points of the lobe such as the eye point as well as used as a method to induce bleeding in the ear

Table 22.**2** Auricular modalities (cont.)

In conclusion, because the ear is unprecedented as an accessible and valuable avenue of treatment, the practitioner is encouraged to rediscover or refine his/her auricular medicine skills not only for easy and effective patient care but for treatment that can alleviate much disharmony and suffering.

Reference

1. Abbate S. *Chinese Auricular Acupuncture*. Boca Raton, FL: CRC Press; 2004.

23 The Ancient Use of ST-36 (*Zu San Li*) with Different Needle Techniques and Point Combinations

As practitioners of Oriental medicine, we know that acupuncture points are a vortex of physiological activity that govern certain body parts. These points may have certain elemental energies; for instance, "water" points, which can add or take away water from the body, regulate water, or they may have domain over the *zang fu* organs or essential substances.

By virtue of simply sticking needles into a point, physiological functions are not automatically activated. In order to achieve the therapeutic usage of a point, some style of needle technique needs to be applied. It could involve the active twirling of the needle (a typical Chinese technique) or simply the subtle but as equally effective positioning of a needle in relation to the flow of *qi* in the channel (a common Japanese method).

In this chapter, these concepts are illustrated by showing the use of a particular point, ST-36 (*zu san li*), and how it can achieve varied clinical effects in two ways—first by the specific needle technique employed, and second, by its combination with certain points. *Zu san li* was specifically chosen because of its multiple clinical energetics and its importance in the clinician's repertoire of treatment points.

In the Chinese body of points, ST-36 is perhaps the most renowned. From a classical standpoint, we know it as the *he* (uniting) point of the stomach channel. *He* (uniting) points are those in which the *qi* of the channel is deeply converged. Thus, they have a direct effect upon the organ, in this case the stomach. Likewise, on a *yang* channel, *he* (uniting) points correspond to "earth" points elementally. This means these points can regulate "earth" energy, by "adding" or "taking" away "earth" energy, for instance dampness. The way to achieve the addition or removal of the dampness is by way of needle technique. A tonification technique can strengthen the earth element and a dispersion technique can disperse excess earth energy. Therefore, we can appreciate the critical relationship of needle technique to point selection. Point selection, of course, is contingent upon the treatment plan, which in turn is constructed in coordination with the diagnosis.

Returning specifically to ST-36, as an earth point on an earth channel, it possesses additional status of an horary point. Horary points have the same elemental energy as the channel that they are located on. Possessing this unique quality is analogous to a "double dose" so to speak of that elemental energy. In the case of ST-36, as an horary point on an earth channel, this makes it a very "earthy" point. But again, it is through needle technique that we decide what to do with that earth energy.

In terms of indications, that is, clinical conditions that are a direct function of the classical energetics discussed above, ST-36 is known for treating gastric pain, vomiting, abdominal distention, indigestion, borborygamus, diarrhea, constipation, dysentery, mastitis, dizziness, mental disorders, hemiplegia, beriberi, aching of the knee joint, breast abscesses, edema of the limbs, difficult urination, loss of urine, paralysis, seizures, asthma (lung or kidney type), duodenal ulcers, depression, and abdominal and gastric illness.

In acupuncture treatment it is rare for only one point to be needled. Therefore let us turn our attention to the use of ST-36 with other acupuncture points to see how they work synergistically, as well as which needle technique needs to be chosen to accomplish those results. Source materials for this discussion were obtained in a lecture I attended in 1988 at the International Training Center of the Academy of Traditional Chinese Medicine in Beijing, China, entitled "Very Famous Old Prescriptions for ST-36." In lieu of a lengthy discussion, and for convenience, this information is summarized in Table 23.1. The practitioner may select any tonification (reinforcement) or dispersion (reduction) techniques that he/she prefers. Standard point locations and depths of insertion should be used and if required, may be consulted.

Point Combination	Needle Method	Energetics	Clinical Conditions
ST-36 and SP-6 (*san yin jiao*)	Reinforce Reinforce	To elevate the *yang qi* To strengthen the *yin* and the blood; for vacuity and cold of the spleen or vacuity of *qi* Overall, the main prescription to tonify the *qi* and blood	For rheumatic disease, *bi*-syndromes, numbness of the legs
ST-36 and GB-34 (*yang ling quan*)	Reduce Reduce	*He* (uniting) point to eliminate turbidity (damp/phlegm) in the stomach *He* (uniting) point to clear heat in the liver and the gall bladder Overall aim: to harmonize wood and earth. For diseases of wood and earth, such as retention of phlegm in the middle burner	Diarrhea, vomiting, nausea, acid regurgitation, *bi*-syndrome, knee pain, beriberi of the foot
ST-36 and SP-9 (*yin ling quan*)	Reinforce both points or use even technique	As *he* (uniting) points, they strengthen the middle burner, dispel damp, and promote transformation and transportation	Reduces edema caused by the dysfunction of the heart and kidney, dysuria, edema of the lower extremities, for digestion with abdominal distention, chronic diarrhea
ST-36 GB-39 (*xuan zhong*)	Reduce Reduce Apply moxa to GB-39 to prevent windstroke	Promotes circulation of channels and collaterals Reduces/clears heat/fire in the gall bladder. A must for any marrow problem. Tonifies the marrow For kidney problems caused by gall bladder fire	Poliomyelitis, *wei*-syndrome Early signs of windstroke such as numbness of hands or hemiplegia Hypertension
ST-36 and LR-3 (*tai chong*)	Reinforce Reduce	Strengthens earth, harmonizes stomach Pacifies the liver	For chronic hepatitis and jaundice
ST-36 and BL-67 (*zhi yin*)	Moxa recommended over needle	Affects the fetus	Difficult labor, promotes menstrual flow
ST-36 and KI-1 (*yong quan*)	Reinforce Reduce	For perversion of *qi*, any *qi* going the wrong way, brings *qi* down	Coma due to anger, sunstroke, toxic coma, respiratory failure, dehydration, makes blood pressure normal

Table 23.**1** Point combinations with ST-36 (*zu san li*)

Point Combination	Needle Method	Energetics	Clinical Conditions
ST-36 and LI-20 (*ying xiang*)	Reinforce Reduce	Both points of the foot and hand *yang ming*	Acute or chronic rhinitis, nasal obstruction due to invasion of wind-cold (vacuity case)
ST-36 and LU-7 (*lie que*)	Tonify Reduce	Benefits and strengthens the stomach Resolves phlegm	Vacuity cough caused by fatigue, deficiency asthma
ST-36 and PC-8 (*lao gong*)	Reduce Reduce	Clears heat in the diaphragm and chest Clears heat in heart and lung. Descends upward attack of heat	Stifling sensation in the chest, dry retching, irritability, belching, irascibility, vomiting, acid regurgitation, lassitude
ST-36 and LI-2 (*er jian*)	Reduce Reduce	Reduces fire in the *yang ming*, clears heat in the stomach channel	Toothache caused by upward attack of stomach fire, headache due to upward attack of heat in the *yang ming*, sore throat, frontal headache, red face
ST-36 and TB-6 (*zhi gou*)	Reduce Reinforce	ST-36 for *fu* organs TB-6 for regulating *qi* of three burners of the *fu* organs	Famous prescription for constipation due to depression of *qi* in three burners and dysfunction of spleen and stomach. Can use for constipation in pregnancy
ST-36 and LI-10 (*shou san li*)	Reinforce Reinforce	Regulates the *qi* of the foot and hand *yang ming* For disorders of the *qi* of the stomach and intestines Vacuity of *qi* and blood in general and in the elderly	Stomach and intestinal problems. Good formula for health Weakness in spleen and stomach, abdominal distention, fullness and pain, loose stools, irregular bowel movement, constipation, anorexia Dizziness, vertigo, blurry vision, weakness of lower limbs, fatigue, hemiplegia, *wei* and *bi*-syndromes, trembling of extremities due to *qi* and blood vacuity seen in older patients

Table 23.**1** Point combinations with ST-36 (*zu san li*) (cont.)

Point Combination	Needle Method	Energetics	Clinical Conditions
ST-36 and	Reduce	Very famous ancient prescription to regulate the upper and middle burner	Removes food retention
CV-21 (*xuan ji*)	Reduce	Sends *qi* downward. When spleen and stomach lose the ability to transform and transport	Severe asthma, improper food intake, abdominal distention, nausea, anorexia, fullness, belching, loose stool, hard masses
ST-36 and	Reinforce	Strengthens the spleen and stomach	Abdominal pain, spontaneous sweat, lassitude
CV-11 (*jian li*)	Reinforce	Harmonizes the stomach. Ascends the clear. Resolves damp Main prescription for stomach disorders and epigastric pain	Eases the chest, chronic diarrhea due to dysfunction of the stomach and intestines
ST-36 and	Reinforce	Main prescription for stomach ulcer	Stomach ulcer, epigastric pain
CV-12 (*zhong wan*)	Reinforce		
ST-36 and	Reinforce	Regulates and harmonizes the *qi* of the stomach and intestines	Wide indications
	Reduce		Chronic diarrhea
ST-25 (*tian tu*)	Reinforce	Disorders of transportation in intestines	Acute diarrhea
	Reduce		Constipation due to disorders of transportation in intestines.
	Retain needle 2 hours for dysentery		Very effective in treating bacterial dysentery
ST-36 and	Reinforce	Main prescription to tonify *qi*. Especially good for *qi* vacuity	Wide indications. After severe disease
CV-6 (*qi hai*)	Reinforce If *qi* is deranged, reduce		
ST-36 and	Reinforce	Eliminates the pathogen	Tuberculosis of the lung, deficiency due to fatigue
BL-43 (*gao huang*)	Reinforce	Strengthens the anti-pathogenic *qi* for keeping fit and healthy	

Table 23.**1** Point combinations with ST-36 (*zu san li*) (cont.)

Point Combination	Needle Method	Energetics	Clinical Conditions
ST-36 and	Reinforce or even	Harmonizes the blood. Checks bleeding	Vomiting blood due to coldness in spleen (failure to control the blood)
BL-17 (*ge shu*)	Reinforce or even needle. Position tip of needle toward spine	Produces blood	For upper respiratory and digestive tract
ST-36 and	Reinforce	Promotes *qi*	Dizziness, blurry vision due to liver blood vacuity
BL-18 (*gan shu*)	Reinforce (needle BL-18 first)	Replenishes blood	Lassitude due to dysfunction of stomach and liver, dysfunction of spleen and stomach
ST-36 and	Reinforce	Decline of *ming men* fire	Impotence, prospermia
GV-4 (*ming men*)	Reinforce (moxa can be used)		
ST-36 and PC-6 (*nei guan*)	Reinforce or even movement	Harmonizes the stomach, invigorates *yang qi*	Stops vomiting, spontaneous sweat caused by *yang xu*
ST-36 and	Reinforce	Tonic points	Premature ejaculation
CV-4 (*guan yuan*)	Reinforce	Abdominal crossing of three-leg *yin*, better than SP-6. Includes function of SP-6. Tonifies source *qi*	Impotence due to *qi* vacuity
ST-36 and	Reduce	Anti-inflammatory. Lowers white blood cells when there is inflammation	White blood cell pathology
GV-14 (*da zhui*)	Reduce Can raise white blood cell count with use of moxa		
ST-36 and	Reinforce	Regulates the *qi* of stomach and intestines	Acute and chronic diarrhea due to *qi* dysfunction
LI-4 (*he gu*)	Reinforce (reduce if due to an accumulation of damp and heat)	Failure of *qi* to ascend or descend	Vomiting, nausea related to the intestines

Table 23.**1** Point combinations with ST-36 (*zu san li*) (cont.)

24 GV-14 (*Da Zhui*): Big Vertebrae—Central Reunion Point

In any practitioner's repertoire of points GV-14 (*da zhui*) should come to the fore as a point of choice for strengthening the *yang* of the body if it is vacant or decreasing it if it is excessive. More times than not vacuity is our most common clinical scenario but both repletion and vacuity can manifest in patients so we should not forget this highly clinically effective point for those cases. This chapter addresses the treatment of GV-14 with the modalities of needling, moxibustion, bleeding, and cupping for the clinical manifestations of vacant or replete conditions. First, we will begin with a perusal of its clinical energetics in order to understand why it would be chosen as a point of treatment.

As a point on the Governing Vessel channel, the channel that governs the *yang* of the body, GV-14 has a role in regulating the *yang*. It is the meeting of all the *yang* channels. As such it strongly tonifies *wei qi* and stimulates the adrenal cortex. It opens to the exterior, opens the *yang*, clears the brain, and calms the spirit. It also can dramatically increase white blood cell production. It is viewed as an evil wind reflex, meaning this is a common area for entry of external wind. Governing Vessel 14 has been called the point of greatest *yang* in the body. Anatomically, it is located on the posterior aspect of the body, in the depression below the spinous process of the 7th cervical vertebrae, approximately at the level of the shoulder. If *yang* is vacant in a patient, this is an excellent point to needle or to apply moxibustion. If the *yang* is excessive, the point can likewise be needled, bled, and even cupped.

Such replete conditions include febrile disease, malaria, blood diseases, neck pain and rigidity, back stiffness, psychosis, epilepsy, seizures, pneumonia, schizophrenia, bronchitis, asthma, hepatitis, and eczema. In replete conditions the point must be needled obliquely upward to the standard depth of 0.5 to 1.0 *cun* with a dispersion technique such as a large amplitude and speed of rotation or with a vigorous lift/thrust needle technique with an emphasis on the withdrawal. Additionally, if there are heat manifestations such as fever, heat in the lungs, and labored breathing with yellow mucus as in the case of pneumonia, the point can be bled with a #28 g or #30 g filiform needle. Quickly insert the needle 0.01 *cun* into the point and obtain one to two drops of blood. This technique will reduce the heat/fire in the body. The application of a glass cup over the point after it has been bled will further expel blood to assist in a quicker resolution of the problem. Wear gloves when bleeding and/or cupping the point and sterilize all equipment properly after bleeding.

When the patient is vacuous, needling may also be employed using a tonification technique such as small amplitude of rotation and slow speed. Needle obliquely upward to the standard depth of 0.5 – 1.0 cun. Vacuity diseases include afternoon fever, pulmonary tuberculosis, cough, asthma, hemiplegia, pain in the back of the shoulder, tidal fever, hot sensation in the bones with recurrent fever, chills, and leucopenia (low white blood cell count).

Generous and frequent use of moxibustion may also be incorporated into the treatment to augment *yang* vacuity. It is pleasant and soothing to the patient and has the known clinical efficacy of raising the white blood cell count. This is an excellent treatment for patients with weak immunity such as those with chronic fatigue, those undergoing chemotherapy, and patients with generalized kidney *yang* vacuity manifesting as low energy, desire to sleep a lot, cold hands and feet, and a tendency to catch colds easily. Moxa may be applied in any variety of forms that the practitioner prefers such as the moxa needle, indirect moxa pole, direct mini-thread moxa, tiger thermie warmer, or indirect moxa burner. Regardless of the form of delivery, administer the moxa for 3 to 5 minutes per session. Treat subsequently according to signs and symptoms. Monitor for signs of heat aggravation and discontinue if they develop.

In cases of severe vacuity of kidney *yang*, abnormal neck pathology can develop—what can be called a fat pad at GV-14. As we have seen, *da zhui* is the point of greatest *yang* of the body. When the *yang* is severely vacuous, what might be called adrenal vacuity, this condition can present as a fatty pad at that point. The fat accumulation is evidence of the failure of the *yang* of the kidney to dominate water metabolism. The mound is water, tied up in the form of damp or fat. This condition should always be treated when you see the patient due to its clinical significance.

With the patient in a sitting position inspect the GV-14 area. The fat pad extends around this point in a round or oval-shape pattern. It is observed visually as a distinct mound. Further confirm this by grasping the area. Do not confuse this with a dowager's hump. Patients who have the fat pad at GV-14 have other signs and symptoms of kidney *yang* vacuity such as excess weight, respiratory problems, loose stools with undigested food, lethargy, poor skin color, gas, abdominal distention, low blood pressure, cold feet, and more. Patients with hypothyroidism (kidney *yang* vacuity) present with this demarcation as well. Patients who have had a history of asthma or bronchitis, or those who have used steroids such as prednisone, may now suffer from adrenal insufficiency. Of all groups, the steroid users most frequently develop this distinctive feature.

Another disorder in which the fat pad develops is Cushing's syndrome. Cushing's syndrome is a disorder in which the face becomes fatter than usual, usually round and red. The body also becomes fatter, and often a pad of fat develops between the shoulder blades, making them look round-shouldered. At the same time muscle tone is lost from the arms and legs; they will feel weak, tired, their skin may become thinner and bruises sometimes appear spontaneously on the arms and legs. The bones become thin and fracture easily. Cushing's syndrome is uncommon. It sometimes occurs in people on a long-term corticosteroid treatment.[1]

There is also what I call a preclinical fat pad that appears in the formative stages of kidney yang vacuity. The texture of the skin here is commonly thick or fatty. It is more characteristic of patients with a lesser degree of kidney *yang* vacuity than the more overt presentation that patients have with adrenal exhaustion. It should be treated in the same manner and its clinical significance is only one of degree.

Regardless of the diagnosis, to treat this problem grasp the area and insert a fine needle such as a #1 Seirin 40 mm subcutaneously downward through the pad. Obviously, do not come out of the other side. Do not obtain *qi* but use a lift and thrust technique to stimulate the point. Retain the needle for 10 to 20 minutes. You may also use moxa around the borders of the area. Apply the moxa around the pad for about 3 minutes using a moving technique. The area should get mildly red. Figure 24.**1** illustrates what the fat pad at GV-14

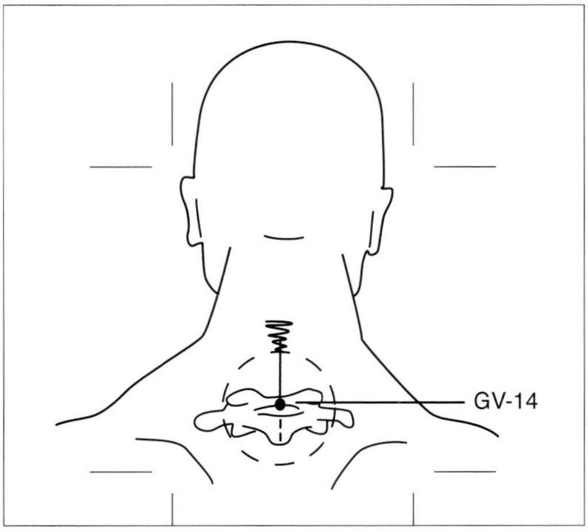

24.**1** The fat pad at GV-14 (*da zhui*) and how the needle placement looks posteriorly.

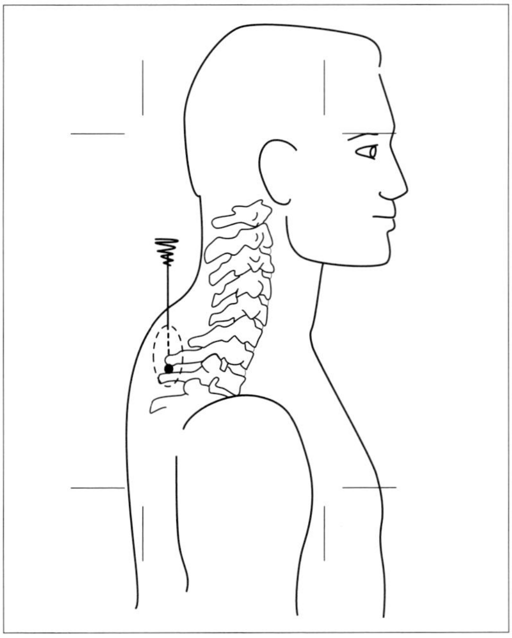

24.**2** How to needle the fat pad at GV-14 (*da zhui*).

looks like and how the needle placement looks posteriorly, and Figure 24.**2** shows a side view and how to needle it.

Supplemental to this treatment, apply moxa to GV-4, *ming men*, the Gate of Life. It is the second most important point to tonify kidney *yang*. *Ming men* may be needled in the standard manner (perpendicular 0.5 to 1.0 *cun*) but the application of moxa is preferable for *yang* vacuity. Moxa can be applied to the needle or other moxa methods can be used similarly to how they are applied to GV-14.

Reference

1. Clayman C, medical editor. *The American Medical Association Family Medical Guide*. 3 rd ed. NY: Random House, Inc.; 1994:564.

25 Modern Use of the Six Divisions: A Practical Needling Strategy for Pain and Blockage

A unique needle strategy called the 'six division treatment' is a rapid and powerful needling style specifically suited to the treatment of acute painful disorders. This topic is discussed in depth in my first book, *Holding the Tiger's Tail.*[1] In this chapter further clarifications and clinical usages are addressed.

The six divisions tends to be remembered more as a philosophical explanation for the penetration of cold or wind-cold pathogen into the body and how its clinical manifestations change as it lodges itself in different energetic layers. Likewise, it has been used to explain the psychological and physical constitutional types that also correspond to these paired divisions.

In this related diagnostic and needling strategy, the use of two acupuncture points to treat acute internal, mental, or musculoskeletal conditions is employed. The points consist of the *xi* (cleft) points of the channels paired according to the six division paradigm. As we recall, *xi* (cleft) points are points that reflect accumulation or blockage in the organ/channel complex. In the six division framework, a channel in the upper part of the body is paired with one in the lower part. The theoretical justification of this as the Chinese say is, "as above, so below." This worldview maintains that energetically the coupled channels work harmoniously together as a microcosmic circuit to regulate energy in the body.

The concept of combining the *xi* (cleft) points of the paired channels for blockage, with its most common manifestation of pain, is simple in design and execution. Before performing the technique, you the practitioner need to select the appropriate division to use. Differentiate the patient's symptoms according to the major divisions involved and then correspondingly utilize the paired channels' *xi* (cleft) points. For instance, acute menstrual cramps can be connected with the liver channel of foot *jue yin* because the liver stores the blood and infuses the uterus. Its coupled channel is the pericardium channel of hand *jue yin*. As we know, both channels are involved in blood regulation and perfusing the lower abdomen, so it also makes sense to use the liver and the pericardium channels.

Using these two points, needle unilaterally with a vigorous dispersion technique, which corresponds to the treatment plan of dispersing accumulation. Insert needles according to the standard angles and depths of insertion using your preferred dispersion technique. I favor fast rotation of the needle in a counterclockwise direction. Because a strong *de qi* sensation is used, prepare the patient for the strength of the stimulus you are about to use, but likewise tell them this is the technique you need to employ in order to bring about the desired therapeutic effect in a short amount of time, which is to get rid of the blockage.

Only unilateral needling is necessary because of the vigorous stimulation employed. While there are various theoretical justifications for which side of the body to needle, I tend to select the side that corresponds to most of the major pulse systems. For instance, unequivocally the liver is felt on the left pulse so the left Liver 6 *xi* (cleft) point (*zhong du*) is selected. Pericardium is correspondingly felt on the left pulse as well so left Pericardium 4 *xi* (cleft) point (*xi men*) is chosen.

If the pain or blockage has a musculoskeletal component such as a sore low back, shoulder, neck, etc., have the patient mobilize the affected area while the needles are retained to enhance the therapeutic results. Needles may be retained for 20 minutes or simply inserted, strong *qi* obtained and dispersed, the affected area mobilized if relevant, and then removed for patient convenience since the work of the needles has been accomplished.

Table 25.**1** lists the six divisions, their corresponding *xi* (cleft) points, angles and depths of insertion, side of the body to needle and some common disorders that can be used with this technique. This list is not intended to be exhaustive, only illustrative of some pain or accumulation conditions.

Division	Points	Disorders
Tai yang	SI-6 L (*yang lao*)—ppd 0.3 – 0.5 in BL-63 L (*jin men*)—ppd 0.3 – 0.5 in	Acute lumbago, declining eyesight, early symptoms of flu, occipital headache, body aches, infantile convulsion and tetany, opisthotonus, stiffness in the nape and spinal column, motor impairment of lower extremities, ankle pain, aching of shoulder, back, elbow, and arm
Shao yang	TB-7 R (Huizong)—ppd 0.5 – 1.0 in GB-36 L (*Waiqiu*)—ppd 0.5 – 0.8 in	Any acute pain or blockage, deafness, pain in the neck, chest, hypochondriac region, anger, rage
Yang ming	LI-7 R (*wen liu*)—ppd 0.5 – 0.8 in ST-34 R (*liang qiu*)—ppd 0.5 – 1.0 in	Mastitis, stomach cramps, food stagnation, *yang ming* (frontal headaches), sinusitis, toothache, migraines, sore throat, abdominal pain, aching of shoulder and arm, gastric pain, pain and swelling of the knee, motor impairment of lower extremities
Tai yin	LU-6 R (*kong zui*)—ppd 0.5 – 0.7 in SP-8 L (*di ji*) —ppd 0.3 – 0.5 in	Acute menstrual problems (dysmenorrhea) or those due to *qi* and blood stagnation, uterine hemorrhage, bleeding anywhere, menstrual problems due to blood vacuity, pain and motor impairment of elbow and arm, sore throat, abdominal distention, edema, dysuria
Shao yin	HT-6 L (*yin xi*)—ppd 0.3 – 0.5 in KI-5 (L or R) (*shui quan*)—ppd 0.4 in	Hysteria, angina, tightness in chest, cardiac pain, dysmenorrhea, dysuria
Jue yin	PC-4 L (*xi men*)—ppd 0.5 – 0.8 in LR-6 L (*zhong du*)—ppd 0.3 – 0.5 in horizontally in direction of channel (upward)	Acute liver problems, menstrual problems, prostatitis, conjunctivitis, any inflammation designated by an illness ending in "itis," hernia, pain in the joints of the lower extremities, cardiac pain, angina, mastitis

Table 25.**1** Six division needling strategy

The six divisions is an ancient Chinese treatment strategy used in contemporary China that gives remarkable and enduring results when used correctly, that is, when there is substantiation via signs and symptoms for which division to use. Mismatched divisions yield poor results. In this case, diagnostic acumen is almost more important than needle technique. The results are also higher if the pain or blockage is acute versus chronic because of duration and the ability to measure results. Try it the next time you are treating pain and the multiple manifestations of blockage.

Reference

1. Gardner-Abbate S. *Holding the Tiger's Tail: An Acupuncture Techniques Manual in the Treatment of Disease*. Santa Fe: Southwest Acupuncture College Press; 1996.

26 Anecdotal Point Usage

As clinicians, we know that acupuncture points have multiple energetics because of the numerous physiological functions that are regulated through the channel system. In this chapter I hope to share with the reader the clinical energetics and needle techniques of some common acupuncture points that obviously have actions consistent with their physiological functions, but are energetics and techniques that the practitioner may not have had the opportunity to explore. I hope that by way of anecdotal recounting, the usages of these points will remind the practitioner to think about the points in this way.

Case Study 1

Late one day a patient called the college when I was supervising student clinic. The clinic was totally booked but the patient claimed to be in dire need of treatment so we told her to come in and we would make room to treat her. When she arrived I had my teaching assistant do a complete interview and perform the physical exam, and after the assistant summarized the case for me I proceeded with the treatment.

The patient was a female in her mid-60 s who was suffering from an acute case of bronchitis that was brought on by exposure to cold. She was traveling the next day to a colder environment and was concerned about her health. Essentially she was coughing, couldn't catch her breath or stop wheezing. Lying down made breathing more difficult so I treated her sitting up. First I palpated the three locations of Lung 5 (*chi ze*) described below. Because of time constraints and the emergency nature of the case, I needled Lung 5 in the tenderest place. Lung 5 was manipulated in a counterclockwise direction with a vigorous dispersion technique and augmented with Kidney 6 (*zhao hai*). Kidney 6 was needled towards the heel, which is considered a tonification technique as the needle is implanted in the direction of the channel. No further manipulation was required. Each needle was retained for about 15 minutes and the coughing and wheezing subsided immediately.

About a week later when the patient returned from her trip she called me and asked what I did in the treatment, which she thought was miraculous, why it was so simple, and why it had worked. She said that it wasn't the type of treatment she was used to, however she was very pleased as she was able to travel without any incident and had not had a recurrence of the bronchitis even though the place she had traveled to was very cold.

Discussion—Point Combinations Lung 5 and Kidney 6 (*Chi Ze*—Foot Marsh and *Zhao Hai*—Shining Sea)

One of the first acupuncture points that a student typically learns is Lung 5 since points are usually taught in the order of the horary clock, beginning with Lung 1 (*zhong fu*). Chinese Lung 5 is located on the cubital crease, on the radial side of the tendon of the muscle biceps brachii with the elbow slightly flexed.

The Japanese have three locations of Lung 5. The first is located 1 *cun* above the standard Chinese Lung 5, the second is the Chinese Lung 5 proper, and the third one is located 1 *cun* below the standard Lung 5. Apply deep perpendicular pressure and see which point is the most tender. That is the point to treat.

Lung 5 is the water point on the (metal) lung channel. As such, depending upon which needle technique is used, it can add or take away "water" from the channel. With a tonification technique water and *yin* are added, therefore the point can clear heat from the lungs (i. e., cool) and nourish lung *yin* (also adding water).

Because water is the figurative son of metal, Lung 5 is the sedation point of the lung channel. It can take away water and decrease rebellious lung *qi* manifested through symptoms of throat blockage, asthmatic breathing and coughing, hiccups, spitting blood, phlegm in the lungs, and fullness of the chest. Locally it is useful for spasmodic pain of the elbow.

Puncture Lung 5 perpendicularly 0.3 to 0.5 in. **Note:** it is forbidden to use moxa on this point. Moxa may shorten the biceps brachii tendon and permanently bend the elbow.

Kidney 6 is located in the depression directly below the medial malleolus. The Chinese also have an alternative location for Kidney 6, which is commonly referred to as "Japanese Kidney 6" because the Japanese use this location. It is located 1 *cun* directly below the medial malleolus at the junction of the red and the white skin. I use the Japanese location exclusively. The needle technique for that location is to puncture transversely and subcutaneously 0.1 to 0.2 in towards the heel (see Fig. 3.**1a** and **b** in Chapter 3).

Kidney 6 is the master of the *yin qiao* channel and a coupled point of the *ren* channel. It is traditionally regarded as the best point to nourish kidney *yin*, thereby facilitating the throat, clearing *yin* deficiency fire and rooting the *qi*. It opens the chest and is good for cold in the chest, and lung problems.

Case Study 2

The patient was a poor woman who was referred to me for free treatment by another practitioner because the patient lived closer to me and travel to her practitioner was problematic because of the patient's pain and the expense of treatment. I did not know what she was coming to me for until she arrived in my office, sat down, "took off her hair," to reveal a bald head and told me that she had terminal colon cancer that had metastasized to several organs. She was undergoing chemotherapy and was experiencing terrible systemic bodily pain as a result of that treatment. She was suffering so much that I was unable to question her beyond her name and the fact that she was dying. Seeing her in such discomfort I did not want to do too much prodding or needling and my general treatment approach anyway is always to use few needles to accomplish the therapeutic aim.

Immediately GB-34 (*yang ling quan*) came to mind and so that became the singular point I treated her with, sometimes with needles, sometimes only with palpation by pressing deeply into the point bilaterally for about 20 minutes. After that amount of time, she would look better, pick up her wig and depart happily until the following week. Even though the patient passed away about a month later as we knew she would, I was always struck by the power of the well-chosen point to provide such deep-seated relief and peace to a patient in great suffering.

Discussion—Gall Bladder 34 (Yang Lin Quan—Yang Mound Spring)

Gall Bladder 34 is located in the depression anterior and inferior to the head of the fibula. The Japanese location is defined as 1 *cun* posterior to the head of the fibula. The easiest way to find the Japanese location is simply to find the Chinese location and then to slide laterally behind the head of fibula.

Gall Bladder 34 has multiple energetics but one of its most prominent functions is the influential point that dominates the tendons and the muscles. As such it is a primary point for the treatment of pain since much pain has a muscular component. Remember that the Chinese character for tendon encompasses the nerves, and ligaments in addition to the tendons, and of course, pain is perceived through the nerves. Puncture the point perpendicularly 0.8 to 1.2 in. Moxa is applicable.

Case Study 3

The patient was a 10-year-old child who was having periodic episodes of bedwetting that were a source of embarrassment and frustration to her. She confided this problem to me so I asked her if she would like to be treated. I palpated Spleen 6, which is indicative of treatment and which was tender and pressed on it bilaterally for about 2 minutes with a gentle rubbing motion. After this *tuina* treatment, without the use of needles the child never had a bedwetting incident again.

■ Discussion—Spleen 6 (*San Yin Jiao*—Three Yin Crossing)

Our standard Chinese location for Spleen 6 is 3 *cun* directly above the tip of the medial malleolus, on the posterior border of the tibia on the line drawn from the medial malleolus to SP-9 (*yin ling quan*). Spleen 6 has some of the most numerous energetics of all of the points with the group *luo* of the three-leg *yin* being one of its primary functions. As the intersection of the liver, spleen, and kidney channels it is an efficient point to regulate these three important and inter-related channels.

Puncture the point bilaterally 0.5 to 1.0 in with a #1 g 30 mm Seirin needle and retain the needles for 10 minutes. Moxa is applicable. If you needle, do so gently with a tonification technique of rotating in a small counterclockwise direction (for *yin* channels on the leg rotate counterclockwise, which is in the direction of the channel).

In summary, while knowledge of the broad classical energetics of the points will offer us the greatest freedom in clinical practices, remembering and sharing your favorite points and success stories with fellow practitioners and students will ensure that many patients are helped. As humans we remember the contextual use of points through cases or stories. Remember, write and share your patients' stories and help enrich the Oriental body of medical literature.

27 The Role of the Heart in Needling within the Treatment Process

In the four techniques books I have written since 1996, *Holding the Tiger's Tail, An Acupuncture Techniques Manual in the Treatment of Disease* (1996)[1], *The Art of Palpatory Diagnosis in Oriental Medicine* (2001)[2] (and in Italian, *Palpazione Diagnostica in Medicina Orientale* [2004])[2], *Chinese Auricular Acupuncture* (2004)[3], and this text, I have tried to present students and practitioners with clear, accurate, and amazingly effective clinical strategies about treating patients with both Chinese and Japanese medicine.

In addition to writing these books, I have taught most of this material to hundreds of students at the Albuquerque campus of Southwest Acupuncture College (of which I am the Executive Director) for 5 years and the Santa Fe campus for over 17 years. Repeatedly the students have adopted these proven techniques enthusiastically and carefully practiced them on thousands of patients with great success.

As beginners just learning these approaches for the first time in class, their diagnoses could always have been more precise, their point locations more accurate, and their needle techniques more defined, yet the compassion, caring and purity of heart with which the students applied these techniques more than compensated for any lack of technique, for indeed the spirit is more powerful than the physical action.

As presented in my fifth and forthcoming book, *The Spiritual Practice of Clinical Medicine*, my premise is simple—effective treatment and healing is delivered, more than any other variable, through the loving, compassionate, spirit of the practitioner. Personally, the most effective treatment I have ever received, in any realm of medicine—allopathic, chiropractic, massage or acupuncture—has been when the practitioner was kind, sensitive, and caring. Even if their technique was not that great, or even if they did not do anything apart from listening and offering a thoughtful word in their helplessness or bewilderment, I was surely healed in those simple moments when another human being reached out to me with an open heart. Likewise, the times when indeed I was most injured and suffered incalculably was not with a needle or an herbal formula, a misdiagnosis or a supplement, although all these things did happen, but when someone simply could not open their heart even enough to ask how I was feeling when it was obvious I was ill.

Acupuncture is most effective when it is coordinated with the spirit of the practitioner, in concert with the practitioner distilling the essence of the diagnosis (what one could call the spirit of the patient), and the essence or physiology of the points (or their spirit). Remember, the heart in Chinese medicine pertains to our boundaries, our eyes, our mind, our consciousness, and our spirit, so it encompasses the highest level of our being.

An open heart is part of the "spirit connection" the *Huang Di Nei Jing* refers to as the essence of healing. As practitioners and human beings, that love expressed in compassion, the willingness to listen, or simply be present, may be the greatest gift we can give one another. Even with technical weaknesses in diagnosis, treatment plans, modalities, point location, and needle technique, healing can still occur when it comes from the heart. This is certainly not to say that all of the components of executing treatment mentioned above are not important, for they surely are, and there is no excuse for never doing the best that we can.

A consistent ethic, which supports life and encourages its existence, is conveyed through your words, your gestures, and your demeanor. Prayer, thought, hope, and touch are all powerful vehicles that impact healing, for they are positive energy that affirms the life force. The integrated body-mind-spirit responds quickly and adeptly to the energy expressed through the heart.

So in your practice, don't neglect to pay full attention to your patient, to respond genuinely to the fullness of their presence even if it is simply to proffer a tissue or heartfeltly to say, "That must be awful," or "I am so sorry for your pain." Don't let all the paperwork, time constraints, how you feel that day, or anything else, be more important than the patients you are dedicated to treating in this noble profession. When you put on your clinic coat, remind yourself to open your heart at the same time.

"Comfort always, cure rarely," is a Western adage that I find as a practitioner to be a good guiding principle, for while we may not be able to cure every disorder, it is always within our reach to extend comfort with the most subtle of tools: the needle and the heart.

References

1. Gardner-Abbate S. *Holding the Tiger's Tail: An Acupuncture Techniques Manual in the Treatment of Disease*. Santa Fe: Southwest Acupuncture College Press; 1996.
2. Gardner-Abbate S. *The Art of Palpatory Diagnosis in Oriental Medicine*. London: Churchill Livingstone; 2001. (Also available in Italian as *Palpazione Diagnostica in Orientale Medicina* [2004].)
3. Abbate S. *Chinese Auricular Acupuncture*. Boca Raton, FL: CRC Press; 2004.

Appendix

Woodlock Oil

Your practitioner has prescribed Woodlock Oil for you. Woodlock Oil is an external liniment used to relax muscular tension, soothe arthritis, and temporarily relieve minor aches and pains of muscles and joints associated with simple backache and general strain.

Apply liberally with a cotton ball _____ times per day to the following areas:

____

____

Caution: Woodlock Oil can cause salicylate poisoning if used in excess. Woodlock Oil is warm in nature. Do not apply to face or open wounds, or inflamed areas of the body. Do not use on children under age 2. For sensitive skin, test on a small patch of skin before applying to widespread areas. If skin irritation develops, discontinue use. Keep away from flames. Do not bind the area of application or constrict the treated area in a severe fashion with a bandage. Do not massage the area after the liniment has been applied. Avoid contact with eyes.

Regal Oil *(Kwan Loong* Oil)

Your practitioner has prescribed Regal Oil (*Kwan Loong* Oil) for you. Regal Oil is an external liniment that is cooling in nature. It relieves inflammation, aches and pains of muscles and joints, such as backache, arthritis, bruises, sprains, and strains.

Apply liberally with a cotton ball _____ times per day to the following areas:

____

____

Caution: Regal Oil is for external use only. Avoid contact with eyes. Do not apply to open wounds or damaged skin. Do not bandage tightly. If severe irritation occurs, discontinue use immediately and contact your practitioner.

White Flower Oil

Your practitioner has prescribed White Flower Oil for you. White Flower Oil is mainly an external liniment used to relieve itching, stop swelling, and reduce inflammation at the local area. It is especially good for insect bites, headaches, neuralgia, and some types of arthritis.

Apply liberally with a cotton ball ______ times per day to the following areas:

____

____

Caution: Avoid contact with eyes. In addition, White Flower Oil can be used internally for cases of sore throat. Do not consume the White Flower Oil alone. Mix 3 drops of White Flower Oil to an 8 oz (235 ml) glass of water. Drink or gargle with for 2 to 3 days.

Po Sum On Oil

Your practitioner has prescribed *Po Sum On* Oil for you. *Po Sum On* Oil is an external liniment that gives warm, soothing relief for muscle aches, joint pain, and minor bruises and strains. It is also used for chest cough and the treatment of toothache and sore throat.

Apply liberally with a cotton ball _____ times per day to the following areas:

____

____

For toothache, dab a little on the base of the affected tooth as needed with a swab. For sore throat, add a few drops to a quarter-glass of water and gargle for 1 minute as needed.

Caution: Avoid eyes and open wounds. If skin irritation develops, discontinue use. Keep away from flames or high temperatures. Not recommended for sore throats in children under 7 years of age.

Wan Hua Oil

Your practitioner has prescribed *Wan Hua* Oil for you. *Wan Hua* is an external liniment used to promote healing of burns, cuts, bleeding, and various traumas. *Wan Hua* relieves pain, promotes blood circulation, and relaxes sinews and tendons at the local area.

Apply liberally with a cotton ball ______ times per day to the following areas:

____

____

Caution: Do not use *Wan Hua* if you are pregnant or suspect you may be pregnant. If skin irritation develops, discontinue use. Avoid mucous membranes. Keep away from flames or high temperatures. *Wan Hua* may stain clothing.

Bruise and Pain Plaster

Your practitioner has prescribed Bruise and Pain Plaster for you. This plaster is for external use only to promote circulation of blood, stimulate healing, and stop pain. It can be used on sprains, bruises, fractures, swelling, neuralgia, arthritis, rheumatism, and muscle tenderness. It is fine to get the plaster wet if bathing. Before applying the plaster, clean the affected area, remove hair by shaving, and be sure the skin is dry. If the plaster starts to bother you, remove it.

Apply to the affected area (bruise, sprain, fracture, etc.) that is clean, dry, and hair-free and retain for ______ days.

Caution: Do not apply to the lower abdomen or low back area during pregnancy. Do not use on children under 2 years of age. Avoid contact with eyes. Do not apply to wounds or damaged skin. Do not apply tightly.

Spray Moxa

Your practitioner has prescribed Spray Moxa for you. Spray Moxa is a substitute for burning dry moxa rolls or stick-on moxa cones. It provides the benefits of moxibustion without the unpleasant smoke. It is used for joint pain, muscle strain, bruises, swelling, and fractures.

Apply *Zheng Gu Shui* first and then apply Spray Moxa on the affected areas, or apply Spray Moxa first then use a TDP lamp to warm the following affected areas:

____

____

Repeat application and warming procedure ____ times per day for ____ minutes.

Caution: Spray Moxa is warming in action but feels cold on application. It is recommended to use *Zheng Gu Shui* or the TDP lamp mentioned above to warm it up. Shake well before use. For external use only. Do not use during pregnancy. Keep away from children.

Ching Wan Hung

Your practitioner has prescribed *Ching Wan Hung* for you. *Ching Wan Hung* is an external ointment used to reduce swelling and blistering of skin diseases, bed-sores, skin cancers, hemorrhoids, sunburn, heat rash, large area deep burns and scalds caused by boiling water, oil, fire, steam, molten steel or radioactive/chemical substances.

Apply liberally with a cotton ball ______ times per day to the following areas:

____

____

Cover with a bandage. Clean and change daily.

Caution: *Ching Wan Hung* will stain clothing, so it is best to wear old clothing when using it.

Yunnan Pai Yao

Your practitioner has prescribed *Yunnan Pai Yao*, a Chinese patent formula used to stop bleeding. For internal use, please obtain capsulated form. For external use, apply raw powder form. Internal use of *Yunnan Pai Yao* is recommended for bleeding ulcers, excessive menstrual cramps and bleeding.

Please take _____ pills _____ times a day.

External use of *Yunnan Pai Yao* is recommended for open wounds and cuts, insect bites, and inflamed skin conditions. Put powder directly on the bleeding area and the bleeding will stop.

Caution: In case of serious conditions of external or internal bleeding seek professional assistance immediately.

The Tiger Thermie Warmer

Your practitioner has prescribed the use of the tiger thermie warmer for you.

Please use over ____ points

______ times per day for ______ minutes. Do this for ______ days.

How to Use your Tiger Thermie Warmer

Pull the tiger thermie warmer apart. Insert a stick of moxa in the clip in the handle. Place the cap back on and make sure the tip of the moxa is in the vented area of the cap. If it is not, readjust so it is, otherwise the moxa will not burn effectively. Take the cap back off and light the moxa stick. Gently blowing on it will help it get going and stay lit. As the moxa burns down move the burning end of the moxa in the optimal burning position, i. e., in the vented part of the cap.

When applying the warm tip to the skin, be careful not to get it too hot. Again, you can adjust the burning tip by moving it within the vented part of the cap. Use light stroking motions or deep sweeping motions as if to sweep away blockage and to open up the channel, depending on what your practitioner has prescribed. A gradual warming of the point is best. Start slowly, move gently, and give the moxa time to warm the area. Going fast can result in the skin getting hot too quickly and cause a burn and also the healing effects of the moxa will be lessened.

Zheng Gu Shui

Your practitioner has prescribed *Zheng Gu Shui* for you. *Zheng Gu Shui* is an external liniment used to stop bone and joint pain, relax tendons and muscles, and invigorate energy and blood at the local area.

Apply liberally with a cotton ball _____ times per day to the following areas:

____

____

Caution: *Zheng Gu Shui* is "hot" in nature. Do not apply to face or open wounds, or areas of the body that are inflamed or hot. If skin irritation develops, discontinue use. Avoid mucous membranes. Keep away from flames or high temperatures. Do not heat up or cover with bandages. Loose clothing is OK. *Zheng Gu Shui* will stain clothing.

Glossary

ashi point	Any point on the body which is painful upon palpation. A shi means "oh yes," meaning it hurts
back *shu* points	Points on the back of the body diagnostic of the *qi* and the blood of the organ in close proximity. Also known as associated points of the back
belly bowl	A Korean-style moxa instrument in which moxa is generally burned directly over the navel
channels and collaterals	The channels and the *luo* vessels respectively that run throughout the body
Ching Wan Hung	A Chinese ointment for burns, scalds, and other skin problems
chong mai	One of the eight extraordinary vessels, also known as the Penetrating Vessel and the Sea of Blood
dai mai	One of the eight extraordinary vessels, also called the Girdling Vessel or the Belt Channel
dan tian	The area below the umbilicus, particularly in the CV-4 (*guan yuan*)—CV-6 (*qi hai*) area where the root of the *qi*, the energy of the kidney, resides
divergent channel	A branch arising off a main channel that travels to another part of the body
du mai	One of the eight extraordinary vessels, also called the Governing Vessel
ear seeds	Chinese herbal seed, semen vacarria, that are afixed to the ear as an ear treatment
essence	*Jing*, a rarefied form of stored *qi*
external pathogens	The external climates or other factors that mimic the external climates. They are wind, cold, damp, dryness, heat and summer heat, or a combination of these
fire syndromes	Illnesses characterized by heat of the replete or vacant variety. They generally have inflammation and its characteristic symptoms of pain, redness, fever, and swelling as part of their presentation
fu organs	The *yang* or the hollow organs
Gwa sha	A vigorous Chinese massage technique performed with a scraping instrument to the body to move stagnant blood and dumpness
group *luo*	A point of intersection of the *yin* or the *yang* channels of the arms or the legs, such as SP-6 (*san yin jiao*), group *luo* of the three-leg *yin* (spleen, liver, and kidney)
he (uniting) point	One of the five elemental *shu* points located in or around the area of the elbow or the knee where the *qi* of the channel is the most flourishing

Huatuojiaji points	A group of points on both sides of the spinal column at the lateral border of the spinous processes of the first thoracic to the fifth lumbar vertebrae
influential points	A group of points that exert special influence on their associated entities. There are eight influential points for the *zang* and the *fu* organs, the *qi*, blood, tendons and muscles, marrow, bone, and the blood vessels
jin ye	The pure fluids retained by the body for its own use such as synovial fluid, cerebrospinal fluid and others
jing (well) point	One of the five elemental *shu* points. They are the most distal points located on the sides of nails or tips of the fingers and toes. It is here that the *qi* of the channel starts to bubble
jing level	Where the combined pre-natal and post-natal *qi* resides. It is a deep energetic core level consisting of stored essence and genetic potential
jing	Rarefied essence
jue yin	One of the six division levels, "the terminal *yin*" corresponding to the liver and the pericardium
lion thermie warmer	A metal instrument used to apply moxa
longitudinal *luo*	A vessel that stimulates the organ complex proper. For instance, when needling LU-7 (*lie que*), the *luo* point of the lung channel with a certain technique, it can connect to the organ of the lung as well as stimulate the channel
luo point	A special vessel of communication between channels that can be used to drain excesses from one channel and supplement vacuity in another; sometimes called a connecting point
magrain pellets	Sterile ear bebees to afix to ear
mai	Channel, blood vessel
master point	Also known as a confluent point. It activates an extraordinary vessel
ming men	Kidney *yin* and kidney *yang* inextricably bound together manifesting as slightly more *yang*
mini-thread moxa	Very small pieces of moxa, smaller than the size of rice grains, which are usually applied directly to an area or point on the skin
moxa box	A wooden box in which to burn moxa over the abdomen or in the lower back area
naganos	A group of four points located between the large intestine and triple burner channels. They are found at the lateral end of the elbow crease and proceed distally, about one fingerbreadth apart. Their tenderness is indicative of the condition of the person's immunity
Nan Jing	*The Classic of Difficult Issues,* written about the same time as the *Nei Jing*
Nei Jing	*The Yellow Emperor's Classic of Medicine*, the oldest body of Chinese medical literature, from 500 – 300 BC
organ-channel complex	The Chinese concept of organ, that is, not just the gross anatomical organ per se but the entire energetic sphere of function that it encompasses

phlegm	A secondary pathological product denser than damp
ren mai	One of the eight extraordinary vessels, the Controlling Vessel
secondary pathological products	Stagnant blood and phlegm, pathological products that are formed within the body itself by dysfunction of particular organs
Shang Han Lun	*The Treatise of Cold Induced Disorders ("On Cold Damage")*
shao qi	One of the energetic levels of the six divisions, the "hinge", corresponding to the gall bladder and the triple burner
shao yin	One of the levels of the six divisions, the "lesser *yin*"
shen	The spirit
shi	Repletion, excess, fullness
six divisions	The diagnostic framework discussed in the *Shang Han Lun* or *Treatise of Cold Induced Disorders* about 220 CE by Zhang Zhong-Jing. It explains the invasion of a cold or wind-cold pathogen into the body and how its manifestations may change if it progresses through six distinct energetic zones of the body
tai yang	One of the six division levels, "greater *yang*," consisting of the bladder and the small intestine
tai yin	One of the six division levels "greater *yin*" that corresponds to the lung and spleen channels
Tieh Da Yao Gin	A Chinese herbal liniment used to treat a wide variety of injuries including fractures, sprains, tears to muscles and ligaments, and bruising
tiger thermie warmer	A metal moxa instrument used to apply moxa
transverse *luo*	A vessel that connects to the source point of its coupled channel. For instance when needling LU-7 (*lie que*) the *luo* point of the channel with a certain technique, it connects to the source point of its couple, LI-4 (*he gu*). Transverse *luos* are used to establish equilibrium between a husband/wife pair
tuina	Chinese massage therapy
Wan Hua	A Chinese herbal liniment for burns and trauma
wei level	The first and most exterior of the four stages, see theory of the Four Stages (1368 – 1644, elaborated by Ye Tian Shi 1667 – 1746), which can be invaded by exogenous heat. It corresponds essentially to the skin and the muscles
Window to the Sky points	Points which assist in oxygenation to the brain, hence often said to have psychic/mental effects
xi (cleft) points	Points of accumulation or blockage within the channel
xu	Vacuity, deficiency, emptiness
yang ming	One of the six divisions, *yang* brightness, corresponding to the large intestine and stomach
yang qiao mai	One of the eight extraordinary vessels, the *yang* springing Vessel
yang wei mai	One of the eight extraordinary vessels, the *yang* linking Vessel

yin qiao mai	One of the eight extraordinary vessels, the *yin* springing Vessel
yin tang	An extra point at the glabella region
yin wei mai	One of the eight extraordinary vessels, the *yin* linking Vessel
zang organs	*yin or the solid organs*
Zheng Gu Shui	A Chinese herbal liniment effective for resolving blood stasis, promoting healing and stopping pain. Effective for a wide variety of traumatic injuries

Suppliers

Firard II Device Owner's Manual
(Therapeutic Infrared Device)
Information about the infrared device available from:
Helio Medical Supplies, Inc.
2080 A Walsh Avenue
Santa Clara, CA 95050
Phone: 408-748-9585

Golden Flower Chinese Herbs
P.O. Box 781
Placitas, NM 87043
Phone: 505-837-2040
Fax: 505-837-2052
Website: www.gfcherbs.com

Information on the TDP Lamp available from Chi's Enterprise, Inc.
5465 E. Estate Ridge Road
Anaheim, CA 92807
Phone: 714-921-1957
Fax: 714-998-6090

Lhasa OMS, Inc. (For acupuncture supplies)
230 Libbey Parkway
Weymouth, MA 02189
Phone: 1-800-722-8775
Fax: 781-335-5779
Website: www.lhasaoms.com

Mayway Corporation (for liniments)
1338 Mandela Parkway
Oakland, CA 94607
Phone: 510-208-3123
Fax: 510-208-3069

Seirin Europe
3B Scientific GmbH
Rudorffweg 8
21031 Hamburg
Germany
Phone: +49-40-73966221
Fax: +49-40-7390211
http://www.3bscientific-akupunktur.de

Further Reading

Abbate S. *Chinese Auricular Acupuncture*. Boca Raton, FL: CRC Press; 2004.

Ackerman D. *A Natural History of the Senses*. New York: Vintage Books; 1990.

Acupuncture. *NIH Consensus Statement* 1999; 15:1 – 38.

Aglietti L et al. A pilot study of metoclopramide, dexamethasone, diphenhydramine and acupuncture in women treated with cisplatin. *Cancer Chemother Pharmacl*. 1990;26(3):239.

AGS Panel on Chronic Pain in Older Persons. The management of chronic pain in older persons. *J Amer Geriat Soc*. 1998;46:635 – 651.

Alexander D. Deep vein thrombosis. *Newsletter of the Ontario Massage Therapist Association*, August/September, 1992.

Bensky D, O'Connor J, editors. *Acupuncture, A Comprehensive Text*. Chicago, IL: Eastland Press; 1981.

Bossy J. Immune system, defense mechanisms and acupuncture: fundamental and practical aspects. *Amer J Acu*. 1990;18(3):219.

Cameron RB. *Practical Oncology, A Lange Clinical Manual*. Norwalk, Connecticut: Appleton and Lange; 1994.

Causon R. *Pathology*. St. Louis: Mosby; 1989.

Chang D, Yeung CC, Chung CY. *Through-and-through Collective Loci Acupuncture*. Kowloon, Hong Kong: Medical Interflow Publishing House; 1976.

Chen JK. Recognition and prevention of herb–drug interactions. *Amer Acu*. 1999; 26 – 30.

Chen Y, Gen L. *Essentials of Contemporary Chinese Acupuncturists' Clinical Experiences*. Beijing: China Foreign Language Press; 1989.

Cheng X. Miraculous pivot. In: Cheng X, chief editor. *Chinese Acupuncture and Moxibustion*. Beijing: China Foreign Language Press; 1999:361 – 362.

Cheng X. Elementary medicine. In: Cheng X, chief editor. *Chinese Acupuncture and Moxibustion*. Beijing: China Foreign Language Press; 1999.

Cheng X. Notes on Bian Que's moxibustion. In: Cheng X, chief editor. *Chinese Acupuncture and Moxibustion*. Beijing: China Foreign Language Press; 1999.

Cheung CS. *Strategies in the Management of Cancer—a Series of Works by Chinese Scholars*. San Francisco, California: Harmonious Sunshine Cultural Center; 1993.

Cheung CS. *Toxic Side Effects of Radiotherapy & Chemotherapy*. San Francisco, California: Harmonious Sunshine Cultural Center; 1993.

Cheung CS. Phlegm. *Ab Rev Clin Tra Chi Med*. June 1996:3.

China Association of Acupuncture and Moxibustion, editors and publishers. *Selections on Article Abstracts on Acupuncture and Moxibustion*, 1987.

Chinese Acupuncture and Moxibustion. Beijing, China: Association of Acupuncture and Moxibustion; 1987.

Clayman C (medical editor). *The American Medical Association Family Medical Guide*, 3 rd ed. NY: Random House, Inc.; 1994:564.

Curties D. *Massage Therapy & Cancer*. New Brunswick: Curties-Overzet Publications; 1999.

D'Arcy PF. Adverse reactions and interactions with herbal medicine. Part 2—drug interactions. *Adverse Drug React. Toxicol Review*. 1993;12(3):147 – 162.

Deadman P. *A Manual of Acupuncture*. East Sussex, England: Journal of Chinese Medicine Publications; 2001.

Denmei S. *Introduction to Meridian Therapy*. Seattle, WA: Eastland Press; 1990.

De-Xin Y. *Aging and Blood Stasis, A New TCM Approach to Geriatrics*. Boulder, CO: Blue Poppy Press; 1995.

Dodd M. *Managing the Side Effects of Chemotherapy and Radiation*. New York: Prentice Hall; 1987.

Dollinger M, Rosenbaum EH, Cable G. *Everyone's Guide to Cancer Therapy*. Revised 3 rd ed. Toronto: Somerville House Books; 1997.

Dundee JW and Yang J. Prolongation of the antiemetic action of P6 acupuncture by acupressure in patients having cancer chemotherapy. *J Royal Soc Me*. 1990; 8(6):360.

Dundee JW et al. Acupuncture prophylaxis of cancer chemotherapy-induced sickness. *J Royal Soc Med*. 1989;82:268.

Dundee JW et al. Effect of stimulation of the P6 antiemetic point on postoperative nausea and vomiting. *Br J Anaesth*. 1989;63:612.

Dzung TV. The curious meridians. *Amer J Acu*. 1989; 17(1):45 – 56.

Editors of Prevention Magazine Health Books. *The Complete Book of Cancer Prevention: Foods, Lifestyles, and Medical Care to Keep You Healthy*. Pennsylvania: Rodale; 1988.

Flaws B. *Cervical Dysplasia and Prostate Cancer*. Boulder, CO: Blue Poppy Press; 1990.

Flaws B. *Something Old, Something New*. Boulder, CO: Blue Poppy Press; 1991.

Flaws B. *Imperial Secrets of Longevity*. Boulder, CO: Blue Poppy Press; 1994.

Flaws B. *The Concept and Treatment of Blood Stasis in TCM*. Boulder, CO: Blue Poppy Press; 1995.

Flaws B and Lake J. *Chinese Medical Psychiatry, A Textbook and Clinical Manual*. Boulder, CO: Blue Poppy Press; 2001.

Fu WB, Zhang B. Contemplation of the treatment of cancer pain by acupuncture. *TCM Shanghai J Acu and Moxi*. English ed. 3rd Issue:57 – 60; 2000.

Gaeddart A. *Chinese Herbs in the Western Clinic*. Dublin, CA: Get Well Foundation; 1994.

*Gardner-Abbate S. The differential diagnosis of pain in classical Chinese medicine: unique treatment approaches and acupoint energetics. *Amer J Acu*. 1996; 24(4):269–284.

Gardner-Abbate S. *Holding the Tiger's Tail: An Acupuncture Techniques Manual in the Treatment of Disease*. Santa Fe: Southwest Acupuncture College Press; 1996.

Gardner-Abbate S. Clinical considerations for the use of traditional oriental therapies on geriatric patients in an institutional setting. *Amer J Acu*. 1998;26(1):43–48.

Gardner-Abbate S. Clinical strategies for immune enhancement with oriental medicine. *Amer J Acu*. 1998; 26(4):259–269.

Gardner-Abbate S. Immune enhancement for oncology patients through auricular acupuncture. *Acupuncture Today*, 2000;1(3).

Gardner-Abbate S. *The Art of Palpatory Diagnosis in Oriental Medicine*. London, England: Churchill Livingstone; 2001. (Also available in Italian as *Palpazione Diagnostica in Orientale Medicina*.)

Gelles W. Qi. *Journal of Traditional Eastern Health and Fitness*. Winter 1993:12.

Helms J. *Acupuncture Energetics, A Clinical Approach for Physicians*. Berkeley, CA: Medical Acupuncture Publishers; 1995.

Hsu HY. *Shang Han Lun*. Los Angeles, CA: Oriental Healing Arts Institute; 1981.

Hsu HY. *Natural Healing with Chinese Herbs*. Long Beach, CA: Oriental Healing Arts Institute; 1982.

Hsu HY. *Treating Cancer with Chinese Herbs*. Long Beach, California: Oriental Healing Arts Institute; 1982.

Kim MC. *Oriental Medicine and Cancer*. Belmont: Seven Galaxy Publications; 1996.

Kirschberg G, Fillingim R, Davis VP, Hogg F. Carpal tunnel syndrome: classic clinical symptoms and electrodiagnostic studies in poultry workers with hand, wrist, and forearm pain. *South Med J*. March 1994;87(3).

Lerner M. *Choices in Healing, Integrating the Best of Conventional and Complementary Approaches to Cancer*. Cambridge, MA: MIT Press; 1994.

Lin A, Flaws B. *The Dao of Increasing Longevity and Conserving One's Life*. Boulder, CO: Blue Poppy Press; 1991.

Maciocia G. *The Foundations of Chinese Medicine*. London: Churchill Livingstone; 1989:39–40 (quoting Chapter 1 of *Simple Questions*).

Maciocia G. *The Practice of Chinese Medicine*. New York: Churchill Livingstone, Inc.; 1994.

Manaka Y. *Chasing the Dragon's Tail*. Brookline, MA: Paradigm Publications; 1995.

Meng C. Current status of research abroad concerning the effect of acupuncture and moxibustion on immunologic functions. *J Tra Chi Med*. 1992;12(3):212.

Nagano K. Immune enhancement through acupuncture and moxibustion: specific treatment for allergic disorders, mild infectious disease and secondary infections. *Amer J Acu*. 1991;19(4):329–338.

National Acupuncture Foundation. *Clean Needle Technique Manual for Acupuncturists* 5th ed. Washington, DC: National Acupuncture Foundation; 1997.

Norris C. *Acupuncture Treatment of Musculoskeletal Conditions*. Oxford, England: Butterworth Heinemen; 2001.

Ornstein RSD. *Healthy Pleasure*. New York: Addison-Wesley Publishing, Inc.; 1989.

Otto SE. *Pocket Guide—Oncology Nursing*. St. Louis: Mosby; 1995.

Pan MJ. *Cancer Treatment with Fu Zheng Pei Ben Principle*. Fujian: China Fujian Science and Technology Publishing House; 1992:2–8, 18.

Pirog J. *The Practical Application of Meridian Style Acupuncture*. Berkeley, CA: Pacific View Press; 1996.

Proctor RN. *Cancer Wars: How Politics Shapes What We Know and Don't Know About Cancer*. New York: Basic Books; 1995.

Reichel W. *Care of the Elderly: Clinical Aspects of Aging*. Baltimore, MD: Williams and Wilkins; 1995.

Requena Y. *Terrains and Pathology, Vol 1*. Brookline, MA: Paradigm; 1986.

Ross MC, Bohannon A, Davis D, Gurchiek L. The effects of a short-term exercise program on movement, pain and mood in the elderly: result of a pilot study. *J Holist Nurs*. 1999;12(2):139–147.

Rubin E. *Essential Pathology*. Philadelphia: JB Lippincott; 1994.

Siegel B. *Love, Medicine and Miracles*. New York: Harper and Row; 1998.

So J. *Treatment of Disease with Acupuncture*. Brookline, MA: Paradigm Press; 1987.

The Treatment of Knotty Diseases with Chinese Acupuncture and Chinese Herbal Medicine. Jiwan: Shandong Science and Technology Press; 1990.

Todd AD. *Double Vision*. Hanover: Wesleyan University Press; 1994.

Van Alphen J, editor. *Oriental Medicine, An Illustrated Guide to the Asian Arts of Healing*. Boston: Shambhala Publications; 1995.

Weil A. *Natural Health, Natural Medicine*. Boston: Houghton Mifflin; 1990.

Weil A. *Spontaneous Healing: How to Discover and Enhance Your Body's Natural Ability to Maintain and Heal Itself*. New York: Alfred A. Knopf; 1995.

What You Need to Know about Cancer. New York: WH Freeman; 1997.

Yan S, Hersh E, Lee SL, Wong W, Loo TL, Mavlight GM. Immune restoration and/or augmentation of local graft versus host reaction by traditional Chinese medicinal herbs. *Inter J O Med*. 1984;1(1):41.

Youbang C. *Essentials of Contemporary Acupuncturists' Clinical Experience*. Beijing: China Foreign Language Press; 1989.

Zhang DZ. *The Treatment of Cancer by Integrated Chinese-Western Medicine*. Zhang Ting-liang and Flaws B, trans. Boulder, CO: Blue Poppy Press; 1989.

Zhang YQ. *ECIWO Biology and Medicine – A New Theory of Conquering Cancer.* Neimenggu: Neimenggu People's Press; 1987.

Zhao RJ. Paradoxes in cancer treatment – and the light in this black hole. *Tra Chi Med World*. April 2000;(2): 8, 9, 30–31.

Zheijang College of Traditional Medicine: *A Handbook of Traditional Chinese Gynecology*. Boulder, CO: Blue Poppy Press; 1987.

Zhu CH. *Clinical Handbook of Chinese Prepared Medicines*. Brookline: Paradigm Publications; 1989.

Note: *The author's last name was Gardner-Abbate but is now just Abbate.

Subject Index

B

C